a LANGE medical book

CURRENT
ESSENTIALS
ORTHOPEDICS

Harry B. Skinner, MD, PhD
Emeritus Professor and former Chair
Department of Orthopedic Surgery
University of California, Irvine
Private Practice
St. Jude Heritage Medical Group
Fullerton, California

Michael Fitzpatrick, MD
Private Practice
Mission Orthopedic Medical Associates
Mission Viejo, California

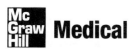

Mc Graw Hill **Medical**

New York   Chicago   San Francisco   Lisbon   London   Madrid   Mexico City
New Delhi   San Juan   Seoul   Singapore   Sydney   Toronto

Current Essentials: Orthopedics

1 2 3 4 5 6 7 8 9 0   DOC/DOC   0 9 8 7

ISBN 978-0-07-143923-7
MHID 0-07-143923-4
ISSN 1940-0802

NOTICE

Medicine is an ever-changing science. As new research and clinical experience broaden our knowledge, changes in treatment and drug therapy are required. The authors and the publisher of this work have checked with sources believed to be reliable in their efforts to provide information that is complete and generally in accord with the standards accepted at the time of publication. However, in view of the possibility of human error or changes in medical sciences, neither the authors nor the publisher nor any other party who has been involved in the preparation or publication of this work warrants that the information contained herein is in every respect accurate or complete, and they disclaim all responsibility for any errors or omissions or for the results obtained from use of the information contained in this work. Readers are encouraged to confirm the information contained herein with other sources. For example and in particular, readers are advised to check the product information sheet included in the package of each drug they plan to administer to be certain that the information contained in this work is accurate and that changes have not been made in the recommended dose or in the contraindications for administration. This recommendation is of particular importance in connection with new or infrequently used drugs.

This book was set in Adobe Garamond by International Typesetting and Composition.
The editors were Marsha Loeb and Harriet Lebowitz.
The production supervisor was Sherri Souffrance.
RR Donnelly was printer and binder.

This book is printed on acid-free paper.

International Edition ISBN 0-07-110524-7   MHID 978-0-07-110524-8

To Renee, who has provided unconditional encouragement, love, and support

Contents

Preface

Current Essentials: Orthopedics is a new volume in the Lange Current series format. This book is strictly intended to provide only the essential points that clinicians need for diagnosis and initiation of treatment of musculoskeletal disorders. For the nonorthopedist as well as the highly specialized orthopedic surgeon, *Current Essentials: Orthopedics* is a particularly useful guide to the appropriate care of patients with the many musculoskeletal problems that are commonly seen in the on-call setting. This book not only enables the reader to obtain the necessary information for a diagnosis quickly, but also makes the clinician aware of the various aspects of treatment that might compromise the end result.

We feel that this book will be helpful to orthopedic residents, as well as residents in other specialties, such as family medicine, internal medicine, emergency medicine, and general surgery, during their residencies or while "moonlighting". We think that the *Pearls* and references will be helpful to medical students during their orthopedic rotation or their general medical clinics. Lastly, we think that the book will be useful to the practicing physician in a number of the above specialties, especially since we have included ICD-9-CM codes for coding and billing.

The organization of this book is based on its sister book, *Current Diagnosis and Treatment in Orthopedics*. Use of the index is probably the best way to find a specific topic. The index has been organized to include the common name for a disorder as well as the more technical name. For example, tennis elbow is listed both under tennis elbow and under lateral epicondylitis. Furthermore, to help with differential diagnoses, tennis elbow will also refer you to medial epicondylitis, or golfer's elbow. Finger fracture is listed under phalangeal fracture, and so forth.

We are indebted to the University of California, Irvine residents, who helped shape the general viewpoint of the book and contributed the clinical pearls that have been helpful to clinicians who are not experienced orthopedists. Our thanks to the following participants:

Brandon Bryant	Brinceton Phipps
Sunny Cheung	Alexandre Rasouli
Matthew Diltz	Keri Reese
Paul Dinh	Kasra Rowshan
Kier Ecklund	Kenneth Seiber
Jeffrey Gates	Jeremy Smith
Robert Grumet	Amy Steinhoff
Gareth Hammond	John Udall
Jason Hofer	George Wahba
Mario Luna	Kenneth Wilkens

We also want to thank the editors at McGraw-Hill for their assistance in putting this book together. They particularly deserve kudos for their patience in waiting for this book.

Harry B. Skinner, MD, PhD
Michael Fitzpatrick, MD

1

Traumatic Injuries

Arthrotomy, Traumatic

ICD-9: 840–847

- Essentials of Diagnosis
  - Traumatic arthrotomy (opening into a joint) is more serious than a simple laceration
  - Because articular cartilage can be irreversibly damaged by bacteria, and the joint environment is limited in its ability to fight infection, treat all traumatic arthrotomies urgently
  - Usually occurs as an "outside-in" injury but can be "inside-out" (ie, from the bone piercing the skin)
  - Needles, knives, bullets, thorns, nails, and bites can be responsible, all with bacterial contamination
  - Commonly, the patient has a history of a puncture wound, bite, or laceration near a joint; alternatively, an open fracture into or adjacent to a joint
  - Compromise of joint sterility may be obvious

- Differential Diagnosis
  - Laceration without connection to the joint

- Treatment
  - The cornerstone of treatment is to ensure the joint is sterile; secondarily, necrotic tissue that may be a nidus for infection must be removed
  - Formal arthrotomy is standard treatment; traumatic arthrotomy may be used for debridement if it has occurred in a convenient place and allows adequate access to the joint
  - Use adequate irrigation to minimize bacterial burden; in more subtle arthrotomies, a standard incision or an arthroscopy may be used to debride the joint
  - Surfactants and antiseptics that are used in open fractures may not be suitable for care of hyaline cartilage contamination
  - If infection is subacute or chronic, include a thorough synovectomy in the surgical debridement

- Pearl

If uncertain whether a joint communicates with a laceration or open fracture, inject 50 cc of saline with methylene blue into the joint from an uninjured area. If dye appears at the laceration site, the sterility of the joint has been compromised.

Reference

Anglen JO: Wound irrigation in musculoskeletal injury. J Am Acad Orthop Surg 2001;9:219. [PMID: 11476531]

Classification of Open Fractures

ICD-9: XXX.XX + 0.10, where XXX.XX is the code
for the closed fracture

- ■ Essentials of Diagnosis
  - • Definition: fractures that involve exposure of bone to the outside environment through a traumatic wound (formerly termed *compound fractures*)
  - • Classification (Gustillo and Anderson):

Type	Wound Size	Contamination	Tissue Trauma	Fractures
I	1 cm	Clean	Minimal	Simple
II	>1 cm	Moderate	Moderate	Comminuted
IIIa	>10 cm	High	Severe, crush	Complex
IIIb	>10 cm	High	Tissue loss	Complex
IIIc	>10 cm	High	Vascular injury	Complex

  - • Diagnosis is based on visualization of bone through a wound, along with corresponding radiographs confirming a fracture
  - • Look for fracture hematoma: bone marrow bleeding from an open fracture wound, distinctive for its visibly high content of fat globules

- ■ Differential Diagnosis
  - • Closed fractures
  - • Associated trauma, lacerations

- ■ Treatment
  - • Debride fracture with remove devitalized tissue within 4–8 h, then every 48–72 h until definitive skeletal stabilization and soft tissue coverage is obtained
  - • Begin antibiotic prophylaxis immediately: give a first-generation cephalosporin for all wounds and an aminoglycoside for 3 days; for grossly contaminated wounds associated with a farm setting or with vascular injuries, add ampicillin or penicillin to cover anaerobes
  - • Tetanus prophylaxis
  - • Operative cultures are not generally useful in acute stages
  - • Always suspect additional injury; perform a thorough secondary exam on all patients with open fractures

- ■ Pearl

Tobacco use increases the risk of infection.

References

Stewart DG Jr, et al.: Open fractures in children. Principles of evaluation and management. J Bone Joint Surg Am 2005;87:2784. [PMID: 16322632]

Zalavras CG, et al.: Management of open fractures. Infect Dis Clin North Am 2005;19:915. [PMID: 16297739]

Mangled Extremity Severity Score (MESS)

ICD-9: not applicable

- Essentials of Diagnosis
  - Many classification systems exist; MESS is used most often
  - Evaluates energy of injury, time of ischemia, presence of shock, and age of patient
  - Value of 4 is 100% sensitive; value of 7 is 100% specific and predictive of amputation
  - Insensate foot at time of presentation is not an indication for amputation; 55% of salvaged extremities show normal sensation 2 y after salvage
  - Low- to very high-energy damage to extremity: 1–4 points
  - Limb ischemia (normal perfusion to cool, paralyzed, insensate limb): 1–3 points
  - Shock (systolic blood pressure >90 mm Hg, transient hypotension, persistent hypotension): 0–3 points
  - Age: <30, 0 points; 30–50, 1 point; >50, 2 points
  - MESS scores >7–8 are predictive of amputation

- Differential Diagnosis
  - Open fracture, type III

- Treatment
  - Treatment of the mangled extremity depends on presence and severity of other injuries, as well as age of patient
  - Classification systems serve as a guide to treatment and outcome, but are not rigid rules; each patient should be evaluated individually in the context of his or her injuries

- Pearl

An insensate foot at presentation is not an indication for amputation. Evaluate upper extremities more conservatively, because amputation outcomes are not as good as for lower extremities.

References

Bosse MJ, et al.: The insensate foot following severe lower extremity trauma: an indication for amputation? J Bone Joint Surg Am 2005;87:2601. [PMID: 16322607]

MacKenzie EJ, Bosse MJ: Factors influencing outcome following limb-threatening lower limb trauma: lessons learned from the Lower Extremity Assessment Project (LEAP). J Am Acad Orthop Surg 2006;14:S205. [PMID: 17003200]

MacKenzie EJ, et al.: Functional outcomes following trauma-related lower extremity amputation. J Bone Joint Surg Am 2004;86:1636. [PMID: 15292410]

Compartment Syndrome

ICD-9: 729.81

- ■ Essentials of Diagnosis
  - Increased pressure in an enclosed osteofascial space that inhibits capillary perfusion necessary for tissue viability
  - Causes: intracompartmental hemorrhage from fracture, swelling, reperfusion injury, or arteriovenous fistula; constricting cast or garment; excessive tension from a surgical fascial closure
  - Clinical signs ("5 Ps"): excessive Pain with palpation or passive muscle motion; Paresthesias; Pallor; in late stages, Pulselessness and Paralysis
  - Pain with passive range of motion of the joints distally is the most sensitive early sign of elevated compartment pressure
  - Obtunded patients: compartment pressures must be tested if compartments appear tense or full; assess by inserting a commercial measurement device, arterial line, or manometer into the midpoint of the compressed muscle or soft tissue
  - Because the highest pressures occur at the level of fracture or injury, pressures should be measured at this level
  - Three forearm compartments: dorsal, superficial volar, deep volar
  - Four leg compartments: anterior, lateral, superficial posterior, deep posterior
  - Three thigh compartments: anterior, medial, lateral
  - Ten hand compartments plus each finger; 9 foot compartments

- ■ Differential Diagnosis
  - Other significant vascular injury
  - Fracture pain

- ■ Treatment
  - Remove casts and circumferential dressings
  - Splint or immobilize fractures
  - Compartment syndrome is an emergent indication for surgery and requires immediate attention if suspected; delayed treatment results in ischemic contracture or limb loss
  - Perform fasciotomies for patients with compartment pressures >40 mm Hg from diastolic blood pressure and in all obtunded patients

- ■ Pearl

Compartment syndrome can be masked by regional anesthesia and analgesia.

Reference

Prayson MJ, et al.: Baseline compartment pressure measurements in isolated lower extremity fractures without clinical compartment syndromes. J Trauma 2006;60:1037. [PMID: 16688067]

Fatigue (Stress) Fracture

ICD-9: 733.93–733.95

- ■ Essentials of Diagnosis
  - Common overuse injury in athletes, caused by repetition of low forces over a long period
  - May occur in any bone; seen commonly in the foot and tibia ("shin bones"), rarely in the upper extremity
  - History of new–onset or increased activity over weeks or months; the significance of activity change must be interpreted in light of the patient's baseline activity and bone quality
  - Associated with the "female athlete triad" (amenorrhea, eating disorders, and osteoporosis)
  - Tenderness to palpation at the fracture site
  - Radiographs usually do not show a stress fracture acutely but may eventually show evidence of bone healing around the site
  - Order MRI or bone scan to confirm the diagnosis or for further evaluation if symptoms do not resolve with treatment

- ■ Differential Diagnosis
  - Strains, sprains, or contusions
  - Delayed-onset muscle soreness
  - Tumors of bone, especially osteoid osteomas
  - Shin splints
  - Exertion-related compartment syndrome
  - Referred pain from the spine

- ■ Treatment
  - Best treatment (almost always): resting the injured extremity
  - If there is no evidence the stress fracture may displace, avoiding the overuse activity may be sufficient treatment; if displacement is a concern, weight bearing should be avoided (ie, by use of crutches); a cast may also be placed
  - Stress fractures on the compression side of a bone (eg, medial femoral neck) can often be treated with limited weight bearing; those on the tension side (eg, lateral femoral neck) are prone to displace with weight bearing and often need surgical fixation
  - NSAIDs are used frequently but may inhibit bone formation; ice or interferential current also may be used

- ■ Pearl

One rule of thumb is, "if there's pain, don't do it" (eg, if jogging causes pain at the stress fracture, do not jog).

Reference

Murray SR, et al.: High-risk stress fractures: pathogenesis, evaluation, and treatment. Compr Ther 2006;32:20. [PMID: 16785578]

Heterotopic Bone Formation

ICD-9: 728.1

- **Essentials of Diagnosis**
  - Heterotopic ossification (HO) is a potential end result of injury to a soft tissue structure in which bone forms where it would normally not form; muscles are common sites of ossification after contusion (myositis ossificans)
  - HO occurs after as many as 10% of trauma cases
  - Heterotopic bone formation tends to appear 2–4 wk postinjury; exception: in traumatic brain injury, HO typically occurs 1–2 mo later
  - History of contusion is important as myositis ossificans has radiographic and histologic similarities to osteogenic sarcoma
  - Palpable, firm mass; some tenderness, depending on maturity; joint motion is frequently reduced
  - Radiographic findings may look like osteosarcoma
  - Ossification can also occur in ligaments (eg, medial collateral ligament of the knee: Pellegrini-Stieda syndrome)

- **Differential Diagnosis**
  - Post-traumatic joint contracture
  - Osteosarcoma

- **Treatment**
  - Treatment of contusion: activity modification and passive range of motion exercises
  - Heterotopic bone formation should not be treated unless it inhibits function because of unremitting pain
  - Most experts recommend delay in excision of heterotopic bone because early intervention may exacerbate formation; after excision, prophylaxis for recurrence consists of indomethacin, 75 mg PO twice daily for 6 wk, or radiation, 700 Gy, locally
  - Some experts advocate prophylaxis in high-risk patients (ie, with head trauma, hip and pelvis trauma, elbow fractures)

- **Pearl**

Angiography and gallium scans can help in differentiating myositis ossificans from osteosarcoma.

Reference

Vanden Bossche L, Vanderstraeten G: Heterotopic ossification: a review. J Rehabil Med 2005;37:129. [PMID: 16040468]

Lunate & Perilunate Dislocations

ICD-9: 833.03 Closed; 833.13 Open

- ■ Essentials of Diagnosis
  - High-energy trauma pushes the hand into dorsiflexion, ulnar deviation, and intercarpal supination
  - Perilunate dislocation: the carpus dislocates, leaving the lunate in place
  - Transscaphoid perilunate dislocation: the scaphoid is fractured, and the proximal pole stays with the lunate
  - Lunate dislocation: the lunate is dislocated volarly, and the remaining carpus maintains its relation to the radius
  - History of major trauma to the hand
  - The hand is swollen, deformed, and tender to palpation; the median nerve may be compromised

- ■ Differential Diagnosis
  - Lunate dislocation
  - Perilunate dislocation
  - Transscaphoid perilunate dislocation

- ■ Treatment
  - These injuries are sometimes missed in patients with multiple trauma; when they present late, treatment is difficult and may require proximal row carpectomy or other reconstruction
  - The acute injury should undergo closed reduction and casting if an anatomic reduction is obtained; otherwise, open treatment and ligament repair with pinning may be indicated
  - Scaphoid fractures require reduction if displaced

- ■ Pearl

The diagnosis is missed in as many as 25% of cases, and vigilance is required to carefully review radiographs of patients with high-energy trauma and swollen wrists. Lunate osteonecrosis is a possible outcome.

Reference

Cheng CY, et al.: Concurrent scaphoid fracture with scapholunate ligament rupture. Acta Orthop Belg 2004;70:485. [PMID: 15587040]

Distal Radius Fracture (Colles, Smith, Barton)

ICD-9: 813.41

- **Essentials of Diagnosis**
  - Colles: volar angulation, distal radius displaced dorsally; "silver fork" deformity
  - Smith (reverse Colles): dorsal angulation; distal radius is displaced volarly
  - Barton: intra-articular fracture with dorsal or volar dislocation of the carpus with the distal fragment of the radius
  - Classification: eponyms are giving way to more useful classifications associated with treatment, but none is comprehensive or universal
  - Fracture occurs after a fall, often on an outstretched hand; incidence increases with age
  - Pain, swelling, and localized tenderness
  - Radiographs are diagnostic

- **Differential Diagnosis**
  - Radial shaft fracture
  - Distal ulna fracture
  - Lunate and perilunate dislocations
  - Scaphoid fractures

- **Treatment**
  - Nondisplaced fractures can be treated with cast immobilization for 6 wk
  - Treatment of displaced fractures is influenced by the fracture pattern and patient factors: age, bone quality, handedness, functional level
  - Closed reduction, pinning, and external fixation can be used to treat many displaced fractures; intra-articular fractures are best treated with plate and screw internal fixation

- **Pearl**

These fractures improve over time, and the final result of treatment is not apparent until 1 y after the fracture.

References

Atroshi I, et al.: Wrist-bridging versus non-bridging external fixation for displaced distal radius fractures: a randomized assessor-blind clinical trial of 38 patients followed for 1 year. Acta Orthop 2006;77:445. [PMID: 16819684]

Bong MR, et al.: A comparison of immediate postreduction splinting constructs for controlling initial displacement of fractures of the distal radius: a prospective randomized study of long-arm versus short-arm splinting. J Hand Surg [Am] 2006;31:766. [PMID: 16713840]

Ulnar Shaft (Nightstick) Fracture

ICD-9: 813.22 Closed; 813.32 Open

- **Essentials of Diagnosis**
  - Usually occurs as a result of a direct blow (hence the common name of "nightstick" fracture)
  - Occurs more often in males, generally as a result of an altercation, fall, contact sports, or motor vehicle trauma
  - Presence of pain, localized swelling, and crepitus
  - Fracture of the ulnar shaft can be associated with dislocation of the radial head (Monteggia lesion)
  - Radial or posterior interosseus nerve injuries are common, especially in the Monteggia variant

- **Differential Diagnosis**
  - Fracture of the proximal ulna (olecranon)

- **Treatment**
  - Nondisplaced fractures can be treated closed
  - Open fractures or those displaced >50% of the diaphyseal diameter or angulated >10 degrees require operative intervention

- **Pearl**

Isolated ulna fractures are easily overlooked in the trauma setting. Displaced ulna fractures usually mean a disruption of the distal or proximal radioulnar joints, if the radius is not fractured.

References

Gao H, et al.: Internal fixation of diaphyseal fractures of the forearm by interlocking intramedullary nail: short-term results in eighteen patients. J Orthop Trauma 2005;19:384. [PMID: 16003197]

Goldfarb CA, et al.: Functional outcome after fracture of both bones and forearm. J Bone Joint Surg Br 2005;87:374. [PMID: 15773649]

Ruchelsman DE, et al.: Anterior dislocation of the radial head with fractures of the olecranon and the radial neck in a young child: a Monteggia equivalent fracture-dislocation variant. J Orthop Trauma 2005;19:425. [PMID: 16003205]

Radial Shaft Fracture

ICD-9: 813.2 Closed; 813.3 Open

- **Essentials of Diagnosis**
  - Causes: direct trauma or blow to the radius, or a fall onto an outstretched hand
  - Fracture of the proximal two thirds of the radial shaft may be considered isolated
  - Fracture of the distal one third of the radial shaft is likely associated with distal radial ulnar joint (DRUJ) disruption
  - Radial shaft fracture with DRUJ disruption is known as a *Galeazzi fracture*
  - Presence of pain, swelling, and often bruising in the area
  - Patients with Galeazzi fractures also have wrist (DRUJ) pain, instability, or both
  - Galeazzi fractures are common; therefore, assess for DRUJ involvement in all patients with radial shaft fractures

- **Differential Diagnosis**
  - Fracture of both forearm bones (radius and ulna)
  - Fracture of the radius and dislocation of the elbow or distal radioulnar joint

- **Treatment**
  - Isolated proximal radial shaft fractures: if nondisplaced and nonangulated, may be treated nonoperatively with casting
  - All displaced and angulated radial shaft fractures should be treated open to restore the natural radial bow
  - Galeazzi fractures: require open anatomic reduction of the radius and internal fixation ("fractures of necessity")

- **Pearl**

Nonanatomic reduction of radial shaft fractures will compromise pronation and supination.

References

Kucukkaya M, et al.: The application of open intramedullary fixation in the treatment of pediatric radial and ulnar shaft fractures. J Orthop Trauma 2002;16:340. [PMID: 11972077]

Ring D, et al.: Isolated radial shaft fractures are more common than Galeazzi fractures. J Hand Surg [Am] 2006;31:17. [PMID: 16443098]

Capitellar Fracture

ICD-9: 812.4 Closed; 812.3 Open

- **Essentials of Diagnosis**
  - Axial loading of the elbow from a fall onto an outstretched hand
  - Patient has elbow effusion, tenderness to palpation proximal to the radial head, and limited range of motion (ROM)
  - Radiographs (AP and lateral) are necessary
  - Often CT scan is needed to delineate fracture and assess for other more subtle fractures
  - Classification: *type I*—complete fracture of capitellum in coronal plane; *type II*—sleeve fracture of articular cartilage; *type III*—comminuted fracture of capitellum; coronal shear fracture of capitellum and trochlea

- **Differential Diagnosis**
  - Radial head fracture

- **Treatment**
  - Nondisplaced fractures are treated with splinting for 2–3 weeks and early ROM
  - Splint the forearm in pronation to decrease radiocapitellar pressure
  - Use open treatment with internal fixation if >2 mm displaced
  - Excise displaced fragments

- **Pearl**

An effusion within the elbow joint together with displacement of fat pads suggests either a capitellar fracture or a nondisplaced fracture of the radial head, both of which may have subtle findings on radiographic imaging. Undisplaced capitellar fractures (or bone bruises) may progress to osteochondritis dissecans.

Reference

Dubberley JH, et al.: Outcome after open reduction and internal fixation of capitellar and trochlear fractures. J Bone Joint Surg Am 2006;88:46. [PMID: 16391249]

Radial Head Fracture

ICD-9: 813.0 Closed; 813.1 Open

- **Essentials of Diagnosis**
  - History of trauma (eg, fall onto an outstretched hand)
  - Elbow pain (lateral), especially with pronation and supination
  - Swelling or joint effusion; tenderness at the radial head
  - Mason classification: *type I*—undisplaced; *type II*—displaced with usually one large fragment; *type III*—comminuted
  - Assess the wrist and forearm for pain (distal radial ulnar joint [DRUJ], Essex-Lopresti syndrome); assess range of motion (ROM)
  - Radiographs: oblique views of the elbow may be helpful and positive for a posterior fat pad or an anterior "sail sign," indicating blood in the joint

- **Differential Diagnosis**
  - Capitellar fracture
  - Elbow dislocation
  - Distal humerus fracture
  - Crystal arthropathy
  - Septic arthritis

- **Treatment**
  - Displaced fractures and those that create a block to motion require open treatment to reduce the fracture or possibly to replace the radial head with a prosthesis if the radial head is severely comminuted; resection is a possibility, but function is impaired
  - Undisplaced fractures are treated with sling, pain control, and early motion (ie, 1 wk)
  - If a large hematoma is present, aspiration of the hemarthrosis can give pain relief and aid in obtaining ROM

- **Pearl**

If, due to pain, a block to motion cannot be ruled out by exam, aspiration of the joint and instillation of local anesthetic can permit a physical exam without pain.

References

Calfee R, et al.: Radial head arthroplasty. J Hand Surg Am 2006;31:314. [PMID: 16473696]

Ikeda M, et al.: Comminuted fractures of the radial head: comparison of resection and internal fixation. J Bone Joint Surg Am 2006;88(suppl 1, Pt 1):11. [PMID: 16510796]

Olecranon Fracture

ICD-9: 813.01

- ■ Essentials of Diagnosis
  - Occurs as a direct blow or an avulsion from triceps contraction
  - Presence of pain at the elbow, swelling, and ecchymosis
  - Patient is unable to actively extend the elbow
  - Crepitus at the fracture site
  - Radiographs demonstrate the fracture

- ■ Differential Diagnosis
  - Ulnar fracture
  - Distal humerus intra-articular fracture

- ■ Treatment
  - Undisplaced fractures can be treated with long-arm casting at 90 degrees
  - Displaced fractures can be opened to obtain articular congruity and triceps continuity
  - Internal fixation allows early joint motion and prevents stiffness that may accompany closed treatment
  - Even with surgery, some loss of passive extension may be expected

- ■ Pearl

Olecranon fractures may be accompanied by elbow dislocation and are a much more severe injury that could lead to recurrent subluxation or dislocation.

Reference

Tashjian RZ, Katarincic JA: Complex elbow instability. J Am Acad Orthop Surg 2006;14:278. [PMID: 16675621]

Elbow Dislocation

ICD-9: 832.0–832.9

- **Essentials of Diagnosis**
  - Caused by a fall onto an outstretched arm or a motor vehicle accident
  - Posterior dislocations are the most common (80%), but anterior, lateral, or medial dislocations may occur
  - Ligamentous damage in posterior dislocation includes both medial and lateral ligaments
  - Physical exam is obvious prior to onset of swelling
  - Neurologic and vascular exams are necessary
  - Radiographs are diagnostic and demonstrate any associated fractures
  - Dislocations in association with radial head and coronoid fractures are referred to as "terrible triads" because of notoriously poor outcomes

- **Differential Diagnosis**
  - Fracture-dislocation of the elbow
  - Olecranon fracture

- **Treatment**
  - After documentation of the neurovascular exam, and administration of appropriate analgesia, perform reduction by traction with correction of medial or lateral displacement
  - Test the elbow for stability to varus and valgus stress as well as supination and pronation
  - Splint the elbow for comfort at 90 degrees of flexion, and start motion a few days later, if stable; longer immobilization is necessary if unstable in the reduced position
  - Fractures of the radial head, coronoid, and olecranon make the dislocation complex; stability may only be obtained with reduction of these fractures

- **Pearl**

Unstable reductions of elbow dislocations are rare, and recurrent dislocations are uncommon in adults but may occur in children. If the reduction is not stable, check the radiograph for congruency of the joint as there may be interposed soft tissue. Even a small coronoid fracture increases the chance that the elbow will remain unstable despite reduction.

Reference

Tashjian RZ, Katarincic JA: Complex elbow instability. J Am Acad Orthop Surg 2006;14:278. [PMID: 16675621]

Distal Humerus Fracture in Adults

ICD-9: 812.4 Closed; 812.5 Open

- Essentials of Diagnosis
  - Incidence is increasing in the over-60 age group
  - Occurs after trauma (relatively minor in the older age groups)
  - Classified according to whether the fracture is extra-articular, intra-articular, unicondylar, or bicondylar (Y, T, H, or lambda patterns), or comminuted
  - Presence of pain, deformity, and swelling
  - Radiographs are diagnostic

- Differential Diagnosis
  - Radial head fracture
  - Olecranon fracture
  - Elbow dislocation

- Treatment
  - Some loss of motion is likely from stiffness associated with the fracture
  - Open treatment with internal fixation is almost uniformly indicated for intercondylar fractures; in older, low-demand patients, total elbow arthroplasty is an option to provide good pain relief and early motion
  - Some physicians advocate the "bag-of-bone" treatment (ie, no fixation and early motion as tolerated) for older, more sedentary and medically ill patients

- Pearl

Casting is the worst treatment for these fractures due to resultant stiffness. Treatment should be oriented to achieving early range of motion to avoid stiffness.

References

Kamineni S, Morrey BF: Distal humeral fractures treated with noncustom total elbow replacement. Surgical technique. J Bone Joint Surg Am 2005;87(suppl 1, Pt 1):41. [PMID: 15743846]

McCarty LP, et al.: Management of distal humerus fractures. Am J Orthop 2005;34:430. [PMID: 16250484]

Humeral Shaft Fracture

ICD-9: 812.21 Closed; 812.31 Open

- ■ Essentials of Diagnosis
  - • Deformity
  - • Pain, especially with motion
  - • Shortening
  - • Angulation
  - • Position of fragments depends on location of the fracture in relation to pull of the pectoralis, deltoid, rotator cuff, teres major, and latissimus muscles
  - • Radial nerve must be checked for function, particularly in fractures at the junction of the distal and middle third of the humerus
  - • Radiographs are diagnostic

- ■ Differential Diagnosis
  - • Open fracture
  - • Neurovascular injury
  - • Other injuries of the ipsilateral extremity
  - • Pathologic fracture with minimal trauma

- ■ Treatment
  - • Closed reduction in coaptation splint, hanging arm cast, Velpeau bracing, or cast bracing
  - • Surgery may be considered for open fractures, multitrauma patients, pathologic fracture, and fractures associated with vascular injury

- ■ Pearl

Most humeral fractures (>90%) can be treated nonoperatively with excellent results.

Reference

Fjalestad T, et al.: Fractures in the proximal humerus: functional outcome and evaluation of 70 patients treated in hospital. Arch Orthop Trauma Surg 2005;125:310. [PMID: 15843948]

Proximal Humerus Fracture: Surgical Neck

ICD-9: 812.01

- **Essentials of Diagnosis**
  - These fractures are extra-articular
  - The anatomic neck is at the base of the articular cartilage; the surgical neck is in the metaphyseal region
  - Both tuberosities are in place
  - Presence of pain, swelling, and ecchymosis
  - Radiographs are diagnostic
  - CT scan may be needed to exclude involvement of greater or lesser tuberosities, or the humeral head

- **Differential Diagnosis**
  - Intra-articular proximal humerus fracture
  - Humeral shaft fracture
  - Fracture dislocations

- **Treatment**
  - For undisplaced or slightly displaced fractures, use of a Velpeau dressing for 2–3 wk followed by gentle Codman exercises will suffice
  - Displaced fractures require closed reduction and pinning, or possible open reduction with plates or rods

- **Pearl**

Shoulder stiffness is the most common complication of treating these fractures, so range of motion exercises should be instituted as early as possible.

Reference

Galatz LM, et al.: Outcome of open reduction and internal fixation of surgical neck nonunions of the humerus. J Orthop Trauma 2004;18:63. [PMID: 14743023]

Proximal Humerus Fracture: Intra-articular

ICD-9: 812.0 Closed; 812.1 Open

- **Essentials of Diagnosis**
  - Involve the rotator cuff and occur in older adults
  - A fracture fragment is considered displaced (a "part") if the fragment is separated >1 cm or angulated >45 degrees
  - Anatomic neck fractures occur at the base of the articular cartilage; 2-part fractures are rare
  - Greater tuberosity fractures (2-part) show displacement of the tuberosity posteriorly and superiorly (supraspinatus)
  - Lesser tuberosity fractures (2-part) show displacement of the tuberosity medially (subscapularis)
  - Three-part fractures are 2 of the above parts plus the shaft; 4-part fractures are all 3 of the parts and the shaft
  - Fracture lines can extend into the articular humeral head (called "head-splitting" fractures)
  - Presence of pain, swelling, and ecchymosis
  - Radiographs are diagnostic; CT scan often helps in assessment of fracture pattern and prognosis

- **Differential Diagnosis**
  - Proximal humerus fracture of the surgical neck
  - Humeral shaft fracture
  - Acromion fracture
  - Dislocation (or fracture-dislocation) of the glenohumeral joint

- **Treatment**
  - For undisplaced or slightly displaced fractures, a Velpeau dressing for 2–3 wk followed by gentle Codman exercises usually suffices
  - Displaced fractures require open reduction for 2-part fractures with significant rotator cuff involvement
  - Three-part, 4-part, and head-splitting fractures have high rates of avascular necrosis of the anatomic head (27% in 3-part; as high as 90% in 4-part fractures); endoprosthetic replacement with concomitant repair of the rotator cuff is indicated
  - Three-part fractures that involve "valgus impaction" can be treated with reduction and fixation

- **Pearl**

Late surgery for failed early treatment produces inferior results to those of acute humeral head replacement.

Reference

DeFranco MJ, et al.: Evaluation and management of valgus impacted four-part proximal humerus fractures. Clin Orthop 2006;442:109. [PMID: 16394748]

Shoulder Dislocation

ICD-9: 831.1–831.3

- Essentials of Diagnosis
  - Anterior dislocation is most common, then posterior (50:1)
  - Anterior dislocation occurs with the arm abducted and externally rotated; posterior, with the arm flexed and internally rotated
  - Posterior dislocation is less painful than anterior
  - On physical exam, anterior dislocation produces "fullness" anteriorly and inferiorly; posterior dislocation produces fullness in back, and the coracoid is more prominent
  - Obtain orthogonal radiographic views (very important, especially with posterior dislocations, to avoid missing the diagnosis); scapular "Y" view, axillary view, and AP and "West Point" views permit visualization of occult fractures

- Differential Diagnosis
  - Fracture-dislocation of the humerus
  - Multidirectional instability

- Treatment
  - Closed reduction is indicated, with appropriate sedation and analgesia; gentle traction in line with the arm, using some internal and external rotation with appropriate countertraction, generally reduces the dislocation
  - The incidence of recurrence is inverse with age and amount of trauma causing the dislocation; older age at time of dislocation and greater trauma causing the dislocation are associated with decreased recurrence rates but with increased incidence of concurrent rotator cuff tears
  - Immobilization for a short period (1–2 wk) to resolve pain for patients >50 y and for 3–4 wk for younger patients is indicated; the correct length of immobilization and position of immobilization have not been determined
  - Recurrent dislocation can be treated arthroscopically in many cases

- Pearl

Because the AP radiograph of a posterior dislocation looks surprisingly normal, this diagnosis is missed 60% of the time.

Reference

De Baere T, Delloye C: First-time traumatic anterior dislocation of the shoulder in young adults: the position of the arm during immobilisation revisited. Act Orthop Belg 2005;71:516. [PMID: 16305074]

Clavicular Fracture

ICD-9: 810.0 Closed; 810.1 Open

- **Essentials of Diagnosis**
  - History of a fall on the shoulder is common
  - Immediate pain occurs at the fracture site
  - Neurovascular compromise is rare but should be checked
  - Allman classification: *group I*—middle third (80%); *group II*—distal third (15%); *group III*—proximal third (5%)
  - Generally, group I and III fractures heal well without much intervention
  - Group II fractures are subdivided according to integrity of the coracoclavicular ligament
  - Obtain shoulder or clavicular views (45-degree cephalic tilt), or both

- **Differential Diagnosis**
  - Other fractures about the shoulder
  - Glenohumeral dislocation
  - Acromioclavicular dislocation
  - Sternoclavicular dislocation

- **Treatment**
  - Groups I and III: closed reduction and sling or figure-of-8 bandage heals in 3–4 wk in children, in 4–6 wk in adolescents, and in 6–8 wk in adults
  - Operative intervention is necessary for unstable group II pattern fracture, associated neurovascular injury, open fracture, associated "floating" shoulder, and symptomatic nonunion or malunion
  - Plates and screws, or intramedullary pins, can be used for fixation

- **Pearl**

Patients should be advised to delay weightlifting, motorcycle riding, and similar activities for 12 wk post-fracture to minimize the risk of nonunion.

Reference

Zlowodzki M, et al.: Treatment of acute midshaft clavicle fractures: systematic review of 2144 fractures: on behalf of the Evidence-Based Orthopaedic Trauma Working Group. J Orthop Trauma 2005;19:504. [PMID: 16056089]

Calcaneal Fracture

ICD-9: 825.0 Closed; 825.1 Open

- **Essentials of Diagnosis**
  - Most commonly occurs secondary to a fall or jump from height
  - 5% are bilateral; 10% are associated with compression fracture of the lumbar or thoracic spine
  - Intra-articular (most commonly posterior facet) versus extra-articular pattern
  - Pain, swelling, deformity, and blistering are common
  - Radiographs (3 views: AP, lateral, Harris)
  - CT scan is used to delineate fracture patterns and stress fractures

- **Differential Diagnosis**
  - Lis-Franc fracture dislocation
  - Talocalcaneal dislocation
  - Talus fracture

- **Treatment**
  - Nonoperative management: bulky, compressive dressing with splint, elevation, and immobilization if fracture is nondisplaced with mild or moderate decrease in the Böhler angle; protected weight bearing after 6 wk
  - Operative management (open treatment with internal fixation versus percutaneous fixation) is indicated for displaced intra-articular fractures
  - Consider subtalar arthrodesis if nonoperative management fails or primary arthrodesis for >3-part fractures

- **Pearl**

Ten percent of calcaneal fractures are associated with thoracic or lumbar compression fracture.

References

Daftary A, et al.: Fractures of the calcaneus: a review with emphasis on CT. Radiographics 2005;25:1215. [PMID: 16160107]

de Souza LJ, Rutledge E: Grouping of intraarticular calcaneal fractures relative to treatment options. Clin Orthop Relat Res 2004;(420):261. [PMID: 15157107]

Rammelt S, Zwipp H: Calcaneus fractures: facts, controversies and recent developments. Injury 2004;35:443. [PMID: 15081321]

Talar Fracture

ICD-9: 825.21 Closed; 825.31 Open

- ■ Essentials of Diagnosis
  - Most common cause is an automobile accident
  - Most common complication is osteonecrosis (avascular necrosis [AVN]); timing of surgery has no correlation
  - Presence of swelling, tenderness, and crepitus
  - 50% of fractures occur at the talar neck
  - Hawkins classification: *type I*—nondisplaced (AVN 0–10%); *type II*—displaced talar neck with subluxed or displaced subtalar joint (AVN 20–50%); *type III*—displaced talar neck with body dislocated from both subtalar and ankle joints (AVN 50–100%); *type IV*—same as type III but talar head is dislocated from talonavicular joint (AVN 100%)
  - Obtain lateral radiographs; may need Canale view (plate on plantar surface with ankle in equinus, pronate foot 15 degrees, and angle the x-ray tube 75 degrees cephalic) to check for varus angulation or rotation
  - Osteochondral fracture of the talar dome is best seen with MRI

- ■ Differential Diagnosis
  - Fractures of the lateral or posterior talar process
  - Compression fracture of the talar dome

- ■ Treatment
  - Neck types I–II: closed reduction and non-weight bearing below the knee cast for 2–3 months; open reduction with internal fixation (ORIF) if this fails
  - Neck types III–IV: ORIF with progressive weight bearing after obtaining evidence of fracture union on radiographs
  - Body: difficult closed reduction and casting via traction and forced plantar flexion, followed by casting in the neutral position 8 wk later; usually requires open treatment to reduce and fix the fracture

- ■ Pearl

Hawkins sign, an area of radiolucency visible radiographically under the subchondral bone of the talar dome 6–8 wk after injury, indicates disuse osteopenia, not osteonecrosis.

References

Vallier HA, et al.: Surgical treatment of talar body fractures. J Bone Joint Surg Am 2004;86(suppl 1, Pt 2):180. [PMID: 15466758]

Vallier HA, et al.: Talar neck fractures: results and outcomes. J Bone Joint Surg Am 2004;86:1616. [PMID: 15292407]

Ankle Fractures & Dislocations

ICD-9: 824.0–824.9 Fracture; 837 Dislocation

- **Essentials of Diagnosis**
  - Ankle anatomy: mortise formed by medial and lateral malleoli and tibial plafond, which forms a roof over the talus; deltoid ligament is medial, anterior and posterior talofibular and calcaneofibular ligaments are lateral
  - Lauge-Hansen classification (most common) differentiates ankle fractures based on mechanism of injury, mainly supination with external rotation, supination with adduction, pronation with abduction, and pronation with external rotation
  - Fractures can involve the medial or lateral malleolus
  - Fracture-dislocations are bimalleolar (medial and lateral) or trimalleolar (medial, lateral, and posterior)
  - History of a twisting injury, acute pain, and inability to bear partial or full weight is common
  - Presence of swelling and tenderness at one malleolus or over the entire ankle; pain with motion

- **Differential Diagnosis**
  - Ankle sprain
  - Talus fracture
  - Ankle dislocation

- **Treatment**
  - Stable fractures (lateral malleolar fractures with stable mortise and no medial swelling or tenderness) can be treated with Cam walkers or short-leg walking casts
  - Unstable fractures (lateral malleolar fractures with either mortise widening or medial swelling or tenderness) are treated with plating of the fibula (for spiral or oblique fractures) and two screws (for most medial malleolar fractures)
  - Syndesmotic disruption requires fixation with screws
  - Posterior malleolus fractures should be fixed if the fragments comprise >25% of the plateau joint surface, or if there is displacement after reduction
  - Dislocations should be reduced urgently, even if surgery will be performed later to ensure viable soft tissue over the ankle

- **Pearl**

The lateral malleolus should be fixed first, which will bring the ankle out to length; reduction and fixation of the medial malleolus can then be accomplished.

Reference

Michelson JD: Ankle fractures resulting from rotational injuries. J Am Acad Orthop Surg 2003;11:403. [PMID: 14686825]

Tibial Pilon (Plafond) Fracture

ICD-9: 823.80 Closed; 823.90 Open

- **Essentials of Diagnosis**
  - Intra-articular fracture of the distal tibia caused by a variety of mechanisms
  - Three groups, based on displacement and comminution (ie, from minimal displacement and comminution to severe displacement and comminution)
  - Usually produces significant soft tissue damage, even if closed
  - Diagnosis is easily made radiographically; CT may be helpful for surgical planning

- **Differential Diagnosis**
  - Ankle fracture
  - Tibial fracture with minimal extension into the ankle

- **Treatment**
  - Depends on condition of the soft tissues; can and should be staged to minimize soft tissue complications
  - Open treatment of the fibula fracture, combined with temporary external fixation, can maintain length and allow the soft tissue to recover from the initial trauma
  - Subsequently, the articular surface of the tibia can be addressed in several ways: minimally invasive plates, limited internal fixation, percutaneous screws, or definitive external fixation

- **Pearl**

The most significant immediate issue in these fractures is care of the soft tissues; the second most important issue is the articular surface of the distal tibia.

Reference

Borens O, et al.: Minimally invasive treatment of pilon fractures with a low profile plate: preliminary results in 17 cases. Arch Orthop Trauma Surg 2006;Sept 2 [Epub ahead of print]. [PMID: 16951937]

Tibia-Fibula Fracture

ICD-9: 823.22 Closed; 822.32 Open

- ■ Essentials of Diagnosis
  - Direct or indirect trauma, open or closed (see Classification of Open Fractures)
  - Higher rate of nonunions due to poor periosteal blood supply, lack of soft tissue (muscle) coverage, and single posterior nutrient artery
  - Displaced fractures are usually clinically obvious
  - Radiographs are diagnostic in most undisplaced fractures

- ■ Differential Diagnosis
  - Contusion, hematoma, or laceration
  - Fibula shaft fracture

- ■ Treatment
  - Acceptable reduction: diameter of both ends should appose >50%; varus, valgus, recurvatum, antecurvatum angulation <5 degrees; rotation <10 degrees; shortening <1 cm
  - Low-energy closed fracture: closed reduction with 6 wk in a long-leg cast; serial biweekly radiographs to rule out displacement
  - Cast (long or short) until healed (usually ≥12 wk in adults)
  - External fixation: for open fractures (wound care easily accessible), or hemodynamically unstable patient or high-energy closed fractures
  - Reamed intramedullary nail for closed fractures, including high-energy fractures irrespective of soft tissue condition
  - Elevated compartment pressures or impending compartment syndrome may be indications for an alternative mode of treatment (eg, unreamed nail, external fixation), at least initially
  - Open treatment with internal fixation for pediatric patients is rarely indicated except for polytrauma

- ■ Pearl

The most common malunion is in rotation. Avoid internal rotation and varus.

References

French B, Tornetta P 3rd: High-energy tibial shaft fractures. Orthop Clin North Am 2002;33:211. [PMID: 11832322]

Mechrefe AP, et al.: Tibial malunion. Foot Ankle Clin 2006;11:19. [PMID: 1656445]

Mashru RP, et al.: Tibial shaft fractures in children and adolescents. J Am Acad Orthop Surg 2005;13:345. [PMID: 16148360]

Tibial Plateau Fracture

ICD-9: 823.00 Closed; 823.10 Open

- **Essentials of Diagnosis**
  - Caused by axial load with a varus or a valgus component
  - Peak age is 30–40 y in men, 60–70 y in women
  - Pure split fracture is more common in younger patients; osteopenia results in depression or split depression fracture
  - Schatzker classification: *type I*—pure split fracture of lateral tibial plateau (valgus load); *type II*—split depression lateral tibial plateau (valgus and axial load; peak age: 30 y); *type III*—depression fracture of lateral tibial plateau (peak age: 30–50 y); *type IV*—medial tibial plateau fracture (tibial spine fracture and lateral collateral ligament [LCL] injury); *type V*—bicondylar fracture; *type VI*—type V with complete separation of metaphysis from diaphysis
  - Meniscal injuries occur in 10–47% and ligament injuries (especially medial collateral ligament [MCL]) in 22% of tibial plateau fractures

- **Differential Diagnosis**
  - Ligamentous injuries (eg, anterior cruciate ligament [ACL])
  - Knee dislocation (spontaneously reduced)

- **Treatment**
  - Nonoperative: immobilize for 2 wk, → hinged cast brace → weight bearing at 6 wk → protect fracture up to 3 mo
  - *Type I*: percutaneous screw fixation; possible buttress plate
  - *Type II*: bone graft, lag screw, and buttress plate
  - *Type III*: displaced fractures require surgery; supplement with buttress plate and consider arthroscopic reduction
  - *Type IV*: percutaneous lag screw fixation if minimally displaced; internal fixation if comminuted; buttress plate if displaced or poor bone quality
  - *Types V and VI*: immediate internal fixation, traction with delayed internal fixation, or external fixation
  - Inspect the meniscus during surgery and repair, if torn

- **Pearl**

Instability in full extension in the coronal plane usually requires open treatment; lateral tibial plateau step-off and widening is better tolerated than medial malalignment.

References

Berkson EM, Virkus WW: High-energy tibial plateau fractures. J Am Acad Orthop Surg 2006;14:20. [PMID: 16394164]

Dirschl DR, Dawson PA: Injury severity assessment in tibial plateau fractures. Clin Orthop Relat Res 2004;(423):85. [PMID: 15232431]

Ligamentous Injuries of the Knee

ICD-9: 844.0–844.8

- Essentials of Diagnosis
  - Four major ligaments about the knee: medial and lateral collateral ligaments (MCL, LCL), anterior and posterior cruciate ligaments (ACL, PCL)
  - MCL provides restraint to valgus force at the knee and is the most commonly injured knee ligament
  - LCL provides restraint to varus force at the knee; injuries are not common and usually are associated with injuries to cruciate ligaments
  - ACL injuries are common and acutely present with large hemarthrosis and pain; the Lachman test (anterior drawer at 20 degrees of flexion) is the most valid test for diagnosing ACL tears
  - PCL is the primary restraint to posterior translation of the tibia on the femur and is approximately twice as strong as the ACL; PCL injuries are not as common as those of the ACL

- Differential Diagnosis
  - Osteochondral injury
  - Meniscal injury
  - Tibial plateau fracture

- Treatment
  - Refer all suspected injuries to ligaments about the knee to an orthopaedic surgeon; treatment varies, depending on which ligament(s) are involved and on the needs of the patient
  - Treat acute injuries with rest, ice, elevation, and a knee immobilizer until consultation is arranged; a careful, normal neurovascular exam rules out the need for emergency/urgent consultation
  - Isolated MCL injuries can be treated in a hinged knee brace for 4–12 wk
  - Avulsion injuries should be surgically treated earlier rather than later

- Pearl

Aspiration of hemarthrosis and injection of lidocaine may assist in diagnosis painfully swollen knee injuries.

References

Beynnon BD, et al.: Treatment of anterior cruciate ligament injuries, part I. Am J Sports Med 2005;33:1579. [PMID: 16199611]

Beynnon BD, et al.: Treatment of anterior cruciate ligament injuries, part 2. Am J Sports Med 2006;33:1751. [PMID: 16230470]

Woo SL, et al.: Biomechanics of knee ligaments: injury, healing, and repair. J Biomech 2006;3:1. [PMID: 16271583]

Knee Dislocation

ICD-9: 836.5 Closed; 836.6 Open

- Essentials of Diagnosis

  - Uncommon injury
  - Usually a result of high-energy trauma
  - Can be anterior, posterior, lateral, medial, or rotatory (based on position of tibia relative to femur), depending on direction of force
  - Minimum of 3 major ligaments are torn
  - Neurovascular injury is common
  - Document neurovascular status before and after reduction
  - Low threshold for angiography
  - Associated fractures of the tibial plateau or distal femur may be present

- Differential Diagnosis

  - Proximal tibia fracture
  - Distal femur fracture

- Treatment

  - Initiate prompt reduction with axial traction; if reduction cannot be maintained in a splint or brace, use external fixation
  - Timing of surgery is controversial; some physicians advocate early repair, whereas others advocate later reconstruction once soft tissues have healed and the swelling has diminished
  - Early surgery is indicated for open dislocation, vascular injuries, avulsion injuries, and inability to maintain a congruent joint in a splint, brace, or external fixator

- Pearl

The presence of a palpable distal pulse does not rule out vascular injury.

References

Chhabra A, et al.: Surgical management of knee dislocations. Surgical technique. J Bone Joint Surg Am 2005;87(suppl 1, Pt 1):1. [PMID: 15743843]

Rihn JA, et al.: The acutely dislocated knee: evaluation and management. J Am Acad Orthop Surg 2004;12:334. [PMID: 15469228]

Patellar Fracture

ICD-9: 822.0 Closed; 822.1 Open

- **Essentials of Diagnosis**
  - Direct blow to the anterior knee usually causes comminution
  - Indirect loading causes a transverse fracture
  - Resisted hyperflexion of the knee can cause fracture
  - Other conditions are bone bruises or osteochondral fracture
  - Need to test active straight leg raise to determine status of extensor mechanism
  - Significant hemarthrosis is usually present
  - Displacement of the fragments may be palpated
  - Radiographs are diagnostic

- **Differential Diagnosis**
  - Bone bruise
  - Osteochondral fracture
  - Patellar dislocation
  - Quadriceps or patellar tendon rupture
  - Hyperparathyroidism
  - Renal osteodystrophy

- **Treatment**
  - Treat minimally displaced comminuted fractures with a cylinder cast for 8 wk
  - Displaced fractures (transverse or comminuted) require open treatment with the tension hand technique
  - Displacement >3 mm or articular step-off >2 mm requires surgical treatment
  - Transverse fractures with one small fragment can be treated by excising the small fragment and reattaching the extensor mechanism to the large fragment
  - Patellectomy should be considered as the last possible treatment choice

- **Pearl**

Always test the extensor mechanism for continuity of the extensor retinaculum.

References

Berg EE: Open reduction internal fixation of displaced transverse patella fractures with figure-eight wiring through parallel cannulated compression screws. J Orthop Trauma 1997;11:573. [PMID: 9415863]

Veselko M, Kastelec M: Inferior patellar pole avulsion fractures: osteosynthesis compared with pole resection. Surgical technique. J Bone Joint Surg Am 2005;87(suppl 1, Pt 1):113. [PMID: 15743853]

Patellar Dislocation

ICD-9: 836.3

- **Essentials of Diagnosis**
  - Can be traumatic or congenital
  - Higher incidence in females, valgus knee, shallow femoral trochlea, hypoplastic lateral femoral condyle, and patients with generalized ligamentous laxity
  - The patella dislocates laterally; the medial retinaculum is stretched, if not torn
  - Often spontaneously reduces, so that effusion is the only sign
  - Tenderness to palpation is present at the medial superior pole of the patella (medial retinaculum); may be ecchymotic
  - Obtain radiographs to rule out patellar fracture
  - Rule out concomitant ligamentous injury

- **Differential Diagnosis**
  - Patellofemoral pain
  - Knee dislocation
  - Patellar fracture
  - Quadriceps rupture

- **Treatment**
  - Extension bracing for 6 wk is the best course (poor compliance)
  - Patellar stabilizing brace and early physical therapy
  - About 5% of acute dislocations require further stabilization procedures
  - The Merchant view is essential to assess the femoral trochlea

- **Pearl**

Consider arthroscopy if intra-articular chondral damage is suspected.

References

Arendt EA, et al.: Current concepts of lateral patella dislocation. Clin Sports Med 2002;21:499. [PMID: 12365240]

Beasley LS, Vidal AF: Traumatic patellar dislocation in children and adolescents: treatment update and literature review. Curr Opin Pediatr 2004;1629. [PMID: 14758111]

Fithian DC, et al.: Indications in the treatment of patellar instability. J Knee Surg 2004;17:47. [PMID: 14971675]

Tear of the Quadriceps Tendon or Patellar Tendon

ICD-9: 727.65 Quadriceps tendon; 727.66 Patellar tendon

■ Essentials of Diagnosis

- Quadriceps tendon tear usually occurs in patients >40 y with pre-existing degenerative disease (diabetes, gout, nephropathies) or use of steroids
- Caused by eccentric contraction of the quadriceps (sudden deceleration such as stumbling or slipping on a wet surface)
- Findings: inability to extend the knee against gravity, gap above the patella, pain, and hemarthrosis
- Bilateral quadriceps tendon rupture is more common in patients with renal or endocrine disease
- Patellar tendon tear usually occurs in patients >40 y
- Findings: high-riding patella; inability to extend the knee against gravity (extensor lag)

■ Differential Diagnosis

- Pediatric patient: sleeve fracture of the patella (avulsion of distal pole of patella along with large "sleeve" of articular cartilage)
- Patellar avulsion (renal osteodystrophy or hyperparathyroidism)
- Patellar fracture

■ Treatment

- Quadriceps tendon tear: direct-end surgical repair followed by 6 wk of immobilization
- Patellar tendon tear: surgery to sew medial and lateral retinaculum and patellar tendon end to end; stress-relieving wire or suture around the patella and through the tibial tubercle may be required; graft may be taken from semitendinosus or gracilis muscles
- Postoperative treatment: 6 wk of immobilization followed by 3 wk of straight leg exercises

■ Pearl

Tensile overload of a healthy knee extensor musculotendinous unit usually results in patellar fracture, not tendon rupture.

References

Greis PE, et al.: Surgical treatment options for patella tendon rupture, part I: Acute. Orthopedics 2005;28:672. [PMID: 16119282]

Greis PE, et al.: Surgical treatment options for patella tendon rupture, part II: Chronic. Orthopedics 2005;28:765. [PMID: 16119741]

Ilan DI, et al.: Quadriceps tendon rupture. J Am Acad Orthop Surg 2003;11:192. [PMID: 12828449]

Distal Femur Fracture

ICD-9: 821.23 Closed; 821.33 Open

- ■ Essentials of Diagnosis
  - Incidence is approximately 37 per 100,000 per year (~6% of all femoral fractures)
  - Two demographic patterns: high-energy injury in young men, or low-energy in elderly women
  - Fracture patterns can be extra-articular (supracondylar, metaphyseal) or intra-articular (unicondylar or bicondylar)
  - Often associated with periprosthetic fractures around the femoral component of a knee replacement

- ■ Differential Diagnosis
  - Knee dislocation
  - Knee fracture-dislocation
  - Patellar fracture

- ■ Treatment
  - Treatment of choice is most often surgical correction
  - Intra-articular injuries can be surgically treated with a lateral plate or external fixator
  - Nonarticular injuries can be surgically treated with a lateral plate, retrograde intramedullary rod, or external fixator
  - Nonoperative treatment is indicated only for patients with minimally displaced fractures or those who are medically unstable
  - If surgical treatment will be delayed, splinting or traction is necessary for pain control and soft tissue protection

- ■ Pearl

Of patients with high-energy injuries, approximately 10% have concurrent patellar fracture, 25% have ligamentous injury of the knee, and 25% have ipsilateral leg fracture in another location.

Reference

Zlowodzki M, et al.: Operative treatment of acute distal femur fractures: systematic review of 2 comparative studies and 45 case series (1989 to 2005). J Orthop Trauma 2006;20:366. [PMID: 16766943]

Femoral Shaft Fracture

ICD-9: 821.01 Closed; 821.11 Open

■ Essentials of Diagnosis

- Diaphyseal fractures of the femur result from severe trauma
- Fracture patterns reflect the type of loading that the femur undergoes (ie, bending—butterfly fragments; torsional—spiral fragments)
- Most open fractures are "inside-out" (ie, occur from the bone piercing the skin)
- Operative intervention is required to mobilize the patient
- Tenderness and deformity are common features of the physical exam
- Hypotension may result from blood loss into the thigh
- Diagnosis is based on radiographs that reveal fracture pattern; *type 1*—no or minimal comminution; *type 2*—comminution but <50% of the two major fragments; *type 3*—more than 50% comminution; *type 4*—comminuted, segmental pattern

■ Differential diagnosis

- Fracture of the femoral neck or intertrochanteric fracture
- Supracondylar femur fracture
- Arterial injury with swelling

■ Treatment

- Closed treatment is an option for skeletally immature patients: immediate spica casting for patients <2–3 y; skeletal traction until healing has begun (3–6 wk) prior to spica casting is acceptable for older pediatric patients
- Closed treatment is seldom indicated for skeletally mature patients
- Most diaphyseal fractures are treated with locked intramedullary nails, inserted from either the hip or the knee without opening the fracture site
- If surgery is delayed more than a few hours, place the leg in traction (skeletal) for patient comfort and hemodynamic stabilization
- Apply external fixators for initial stabilization in polytrauma patients or those with severe soft tissue injuries

■ Pearl

Carefully scrutinize the ipsilateral femoral neck radiograph for evidence of an undisplaced fracture.

Reference

Anglen JO, Choi L: Treatment options in pediatric femoral shaft fractures. J Orthop Trauma 2005;19:724. [PMID: 16314721]

Subtrochanteric Femur Fracture

ICD-9: 820.22

- ### Essentials of Diagnosis

  - Fracture (usually comminuted) of the femur between the lesser trochanter and 5 cm distal to the lesser trochanter
  - Medial and posteromedial cortices are the sites of highest compressive forces; the lateral cortex undergoes the highest tensile forces
  - Usually occurs in young adults secondary to high-energy trauma
  - Can present as a pathologic fracture secondary to metastatic disease in older adults
  - Patients present with a swollen and painful proximal thigh with possible rotation or shortening of the affected limb; blood loss can be significant
  - A treatment-based classification system, the Russell and Taylor classification, is used

- ### Differential Diagnosis

  - Femoral shaft fractures
  - Femoral neck fractures
  - Hip dislocation
  - Pelvic fractures

- ### Treatment

  - The treatment of choice is internal fixation; closed reduction is difficult because the pull of the muscles on the proximal fragment causes the fragment to flex, abduct, and externally rotate
  - An intramedullary nail secured with locking screws into the femoral head and neck is often successful
  - Delayed union and nonunion, and hardware failure, are common complications requiring repeat fixation with bone graft

- ### Pearl

These high-energy injuries in young patients are frequently associated with other injuries, including femoral neck fractures.

References

Craig NJ, Maffulli N: Subtrochanteric fractures: current management options. Disabil Rehabil 2005;27:1181. [PMID: 16278187]

Craig NJ, et al.: Subtrochanteric fractures. A review of treatment options. Bull Hosp Jt Dis 2001;60:35. [PMID: 11759576]

Femoral Neck Fracture

ICD-9: 820.02 Transcervical; 820.03 Basilar

- Essentials of Diagnosis
  - Most often due to falls; risk of injury is related to conditions that increase the probability of falls and those that decrease a person's intrinsic ability to withstand trauma
  - Patients present with severe hip pain, inability to ambulate, and a shortened limb on the fracture side, when displaced
  - Tenderness to palpation over the injured hip
  - Hip is externally rotated and abducted when displaced
  - Range of motion (ROM) is limited by pain at extremes when undisplaced
  - Radiography is the first-line modality for imaging and classifying femoral neck fractures
  - CT is the most useful test for evaluating bony injury, but sometimes fractures in the axial plane can be missed
  - MRI is both sensitive and specific in detecting undisplaced femoral neck fractures, because it can show both the actual fracture line and the resulting bone marrow edema
  - Garden classification: *nondisplaced fractures* (20%)—type 1: stress fracture, valgus impaction of head; type 2: complete, nondisplaced fracture; *displaced fractures*—type 3: varus displacement of the femoral head; type 4: fracture fragments, completely displaced

- Differential Diagnosis
  - Pathologic fracture or impending fracture
  - Intertrochanteric fractures
  - Iliopsoas bursitis
  - Lumbar radicular pain
  - Psoas abscess

- Treatment
  - Treatment is almost always by surgical intervention; this allows patients to ambulate with minimum delay
  - Nondisplaced fractures and femoral neck fractures in young patients are usually treated with closed reduction and percutaneous pinning; elderly patients or those with Garden type 3 or 4 fractures are usually treated with hemiarthroplasty

- Pearl

Do not attempt ROM examination without prior radiographs.

Reference

Macaulay W, et al.: Displaced femoral neck fractures in the elderly: hemiarthroplasty versus total hip arthroplasty. J Am Acad Orthop Surg 2006;14:287. [PMID: 16675622]

Trochanteric Hip Fracture

ICD-9: 820.21 Closed; 820.31 Open

- ■ Essentials of Diagnosis
  - Fracture of the lesser trochanter (rare) is due to avulsion by the iliopsoas
  - Fracture of the greater trochanter is due to direct injury or avulsion by the gluteus medius and minimus
  - Intertrochanteric (IT) fracture is a result of a fall (elderly patients); presents as a shortened leg with external rotation; patients are unable to bear weight
  - Stable fracture: has good cortical contact medially and posteriorly; prevents fracture displacement into varus or retroversion when weight bearing
  - Unstable fracture: cortical overlap or comminution; gap medially and posteriorly; femoral head can slip into varus, and retroversion leads to shortening (>13 mm overlap will affect abductor lever arm, causing difficulty walking and limp)

- ■ Differential Diagnosis
  - Femoral neck fracture
  - Subtrochanteric fracture

- ■ Treatment
  - Pure greater trochanter fracture: if >1 cm displacement, use open reduction and fixation; if stable and <1 cm displaced, place on protected weight bearing (full weight bearing by 6–8 wk)
  - IT fracture: treat expeditiously with surgery, limited only by the patient's medical status
  - Stable IT fracture: reduce on a fracture table; a sliding compression screw and sideplate allows the fracture to impact into stability
  - Unstable IT fracture: use second-generation locking nail or sliding hip-screw with long side-plate, combined with limited interfragmentary fixation and bone grafting of subtrochanteric region
  - Hip arthroplasty: may be required in severely comminuted or markedly osteopenic cases, or in patients with rheumatoid arthritis

- ■ Pearl

Hip screw-plate devices have been shown in limited randomized trials to be as effective as intramedullary nails in treating extracapsular IT fractures.

Reference

Parker MJ, Gurusamy K: Modern methods of treating hip fractures. Disabil Rehabil 2005;27:1045. [PMID: 16856070]

Traumatic Dislocation of the Hip Joint

ICD-9: 835.0 Closed; 835.1 Open

- Essentials of Diagnosis
  - Posterior hip dislocation (usually in younger patients) results from high-energy impact (eg, motor vehicle accident, dashboard on knees); presents with shortening, flexion, adduction, and internal rotation
  - Sciatic nerve injury occurs in 10–20% of posterior dislocations
  - Anterior hip dislocation (much rarer) occurs while hip is extended and externally rotated; patient presents with hip in flexed, abducted, and externally rotated position
  - Palpable femoral head is inferior to inguinal flexion crease
  - Extended periods with the head dislocated predispose to osteonecrosis of the femoral head

- Differential Diagnosis
  - Associated acetabular fractures: obtain Judet films (45-degree oblique views to see AP pelvic columns, acetabular wall)
  - Proximal femoral fractures

- Treatment
  - Closed reduction: perform if acetabular fracture is absent or minimal; usually successful for anterior dislocation
  - Time between injury and reduction is the most important factor in long-term prognosis (delay in treatment increases the likelihood of osteonecrosis and post-traumatic arthritis)
  - For posterior dislocation, apply traction in the line of deformity, rotate hips internally and externally, and check stability and congruity of the reduction
  - Open treatment: perform for open dislocations, redislocation after reduction, or widened joint space (interposition of fragments or soft tissue)
  - CT scan will reveal nonconcentric reduction
  - Patients with reduced anterior dislocations can usually mobilize in days, with full weight bearing by 4–6 wk

- Pearl

In children, traumatic hip dislocation with spontaneous incomplete reduction can be missed radiographically, due to incompletely ossified labrum interposed in the joint space.

Reference

Sahin V, et al.: Traumatic dislocation and fracture-dislocation of the hip: a long-term follow-up study. J Trauma 2003;54:520. [PMID: 12634533]

Injuries to the Pelvic Ring

ICD-9: 808.41–808.43

- ■ Essentials of Diagnosis
  - Pelvic fractures most often occur in a fall from significant height, pedestrian accident, ski accident, or vehicular trauma
  - Three categories: anteroposterior (AP) compression injuries, lateral compression (LC) injuries, and vertical shear (VS) injuries; most are closed injuries
  - Posterior ring fractures are revealed by pelvic instability associated with posterior pain, swelling, ecchymosis, and motion
  - LC injuries are usually stable, with impaction of the posterior structures but seldom any complications
  - AP compression injuries demonstrate anterior instability, palpable ramus fractures, or pubic symphysis gapping
  - AP injuries are often accompanied by bladder, prostatic, or urethral injury
  - Gynecologic and rectal exams are mandatory because bony fragments can exit the vagina or rectum, rendering the fracture as "open" and necessitating urgent irrigation and debridement

- ■ Differential Diagnosis
  - Acetabular fractures
  - Iliac wing fractures
  - Sacral fracture

- ■ Treatment
  - External fixation for AP-type injuries with pubic diastasis >2.5 cm
  - Immediate application of pelvic clamp for unstable posterior injuries
  - Sheet or commercially available pelvic compression belt for immediate reduction of potential bleeding space in AP-type fractures; an external fixator can also be used
  - Definitive fracture fixation depends on specific fracture type

- ■ Pearl

Identification of posterior injury to the pelvic ring is essential to prevent associated significant hemorrhage, neurologic injury, and mortality. Hemorrhage is rarely from pelvic arterial injuries (usually internal iliac branches).

References

Durkin A, et al.: Contemporary management of pelvic fractures. Am J Surg 2006;192:211. [PMID: 16860634]

Templeman DC, et al.: Surgical management of pelvic ring injuries. Instr Course Lect 2005;54:395. [PMID: 15948468]

2

Sports Injuries

Soft Tissue Injuries

ICD-9: 840.9 Sprain or strain of upper extremity;
839.8 Dislocation

- ■ Essentials of Diagnosis
  - Injuries that affect joints, muscles, and ligaments
  - Sprains, strains, and dislocations are considered soft tissue injuries; *sprains* refer to ligament injuries and *strains*, to muscle injuries
  - Symptoms: sudden onset of pain, loss of power and strength, bruising, and swelling; an audible "crack" or "pop" may be heard in ligament or tendon rupture
  - Perform vascular assessment to rule out vascular injuries, particularly in large joint dislocations (eg, knees)
  - MRI can be used to evaluate soft tissue tears and ruptures

- ■ Differential Diagnosis
  - Bursitis
  - Muscle strains
  - Muscle spasm
  - Hematoma
  - Cellulitis
  - Ligament ruptures

- ■ Treatment
  - Acute stage of injury: provide rest to the injured structure, with ice to help reduce swelling and pain, compression, and elevation (RICE)
  - If a tear is present, surgical repair or immobilization with a cast or an orthosis may be necessary
  - Treat any underlying issues (eg, hematoma, compartment syndrome)
  - Avoid heat and massage to the affected area (which tends to increase swelling, pain, and/or bleeding) until the subacute or chronic stage of the injury

- ■ Pearl
Avoid nonselective NSAIDs in the acute stage to minimize bleeding.

References

Gabbe BJ, et al.: Risk factors for hamstring injuries in community level Australian football. Br J Sports Med 2005;39:106. [PMID: 15665208]

Levine WN, et al.: Intramuscular corticosteroid injection for hamstring injuries. A 13-year experience in the National Football League. Am J Sports Med 2000;28:297. [PMID: 10843118]

Head Injuries in Athletes

ICD-9: not applicable

- ■ Essentials of Diagnosis
  - Head injuries comprise ~5% of all sports injuries and 19% of football injuries in high school
  - Injuries can be either diffuse or focal
  - Diffuse brain injuries have no identifiable lesion; severity can range from diffuse axonal damage with persistent neurologic deficits to concussion
  - Although focal brain injuries and diffuse axonal injuries can occur in sports, concussions are most common
  - Principle features of concussion: loss of consciousness (LOC) and amnesia (antegrade, retrograde, or both)
  - Radiographs and CT scan of the head are the imaging exams of choice to evaluate a head injury

- ■ Differential Diagnosis
  - Focal brain injury: subdural hematoma, epidural hematoma, cerebral contusion, intracerebral hemorrhage, subarachnoid hemorrhage
  - Cervical spine injury
  - Skull fracture

- ■ Treatment
  - Treatment of severe head injury is beyond the scope of this book; if a head injury is suspected, seek immediate evaluation by a properly trained medical professional
  - Obtain radiographic evaluation with CT in athletes with any neurologic deficit, LOC >5 s, nausea, lethargy, headache, dizziness, or seizure
  - If neurologic signs or symptoms are absent but the athlete sustained a significant blow to the head, perform serial exams and monitor carefully for 24–48 h after injury

- ■ Pearl

Individuals with an epidural hematoma usually have an initial LOC followed by a period of apparent recovery. Minutes to hours later, there is a rapid deterioration in mental and neurologic status, severe headache, ipsilateral pupil dilation, and eventual LOC.

Reference

McCrory P, et al.: Summary and agreement statement of the 2nd International Symposium on Concussion in Sports, Prague 2004. Clin J Sports Med 2005;15:48. [PMID: 15782046]

The Female Athlete

ICD-9: not applicable

- ■ Essentials of Diagnosis
  - • Female athletes are susceptible to a unique set of injuries and conditions (eg, "female athlete triad," anterior cruciate ligament [ACL] tears and noncontact ACL injuries, and patellofemoral [PF] disorders)
  - • "Female athlete triad" describes a syndrome of amenorrhea, eating disorders, and osteoporosis associated with an imbalance between energy consumption and requirements; contributing factors are the increased energy needed to participate in athletic activity and pressure to achieve a lean body image
  - • Eating disorders occur in 22–60% of female athletes
  - • Increased incidence of noncontact ACL injuries and PF disorders is a result of body biomechanics (weak adductor muscles, weak quadriceps, narrow intracondylar notch), and possibly hormonal fluctuations

- ■ Differential Diagnosis
  - • Other causes of amenorrhea (endocrine disorders, eg, thyroid, estrogen; unrecognized pregnancy)
  - • Stress fractures (hip, tibia)
  - • Other causes of knee swelling and pain (eg, meniscal tears, osteochondral defects, osteochondritis dissecans)

- ■ Treatment
  - • Prevention is the most effective treatment of "female athlete triad"; coaches, trainers, and primary care physicians should be educated to recognize early signs and identify those at risk
  - • Prevention of ACL and PF injuries is also crucial; several conditioning and training programs reduce the risk of injury
  - • ACL tears require surgical reconstruction
  - • PF disorders can usually be treated with physical therapy; occasionally, a PF brace or McConnell taping eliminates symptoms; if surgical correction is required, lateral retinacular release and PF realignment are effective in carefully selected patients who meet surgical indications

- ■ Pearl

Osteopenia: bone mineral density (BMD) that is 1–2.5 standard deviations (SD) below age-matched individuals. Osteoporosis: BMD >2.5 SD below age-matched individuals.

Reference

Hobart JA, Smucker DR: The female athlete triad. Am J Fam Physician 2000;61:3357. [PMID: 10865930]

"Stingers" & "Burners" in Collision Sports

ICD-9: 957.9

- **Essentials of Diagnosis**
  - "Stingers" and "burners" are lay terms for transient neurapraxia of the nerve roots of the cervical spine or brachial plexus
  - Most common in football players, especially linemen, defensive ends, and linebackers; 50% of collegiate football players report these symptoms
  - Caused by traction exerted on the nerve roots or brachial plexus when the shoulder is depressed and the head is laterally flexed toward the contralateral side
  - Patients experience a "dead arm" or "burning pain" that typically resolves in seconds to minutes; residual weakness sometimes persists up to 6 wk
  - Muscles innervated by the upper plexus are most affected (ie, biceps, deltoid, rotator cuff, rhomboids)
  - Cervical spine evaluation is paramount—it should be nonpainful to palpation with pain-free range of motion; if not, radiographic evaluation is needed

- **Differential Diagnosis**
  - Head injury
  - Cervical spine injury
  - "Spear tackler's" spine (cervical spondylosis and stenosis caused by repetitive axial loads or flexion injuries to the cervical spine)

- **Treatment**
  - If symptoms do not resolve quickly, an evaluation with plain radiographs is recommended; MRI may also be needed
  - If neurologic deficits other than arm pain are noted, neurologic and radiographic evaluations are needed
  - If the athlete has recurrent "stingers," obtain radiographic evaluation for cervical stenosis (congenital or developmental)
  - If symptoms resolve quickly, neurologic exam is normal, and cervical spine is nontender, the athlete may return to play

- **Pearl**

The Torg ratio is the ratio of spinal canal distance (ie, from midpoint of posterior aspect of vertebral body to spinolaminar line) to AP width of the vertebral body, seen on a lateral radiograph. A ratio <0.8 indicates cervical stenosis.

Reference

Torg JS, et al.: Injuries to the cervical spine in American football players. J Bone Joint Surg Am 2002;84:112. [PMID: 11792789]

Sternoclavicular Joint Injury

ICD-9: 839.61

- **Essentials of Diagnosis**
  - History of a blow to the point of the shoulder (anterior dislocation) or direct blow to the clavicle in an anterior-to-posterior direction (posterior dislocation); anterior dislocation is more common
  - Injury classification is based on degree of subluxation and dislocation: *first-degree*—incomplete rupture of the costoclavicular and sternoclavicular ligaments; *second-degree*—rupture of sternoclavicular ligaments and partial tear of costoclavicular ligaments; *third-degree*—complete tear of both ligaments with associated dislocation
  - Oblique radiographic views of the joint can show direction and extent of subluxation and dislocation but may be difficult to interpret; CT imaging can help confirm the diagnosis

- **Differential Diagnosis**
  - Clavicular fracture
  - Fracture through the physis in patients <24 y
  - Fractured sternum
  - Fractured ribs

- **Treatment**
  - Anterior dislocations are not treated operatively; closed reduction can be attempted; treat in a sling
  - Posterior dislocation can be dangerous, because it may impinge on vessels, trachea, esophagus, and thoracic duct; therefore, treatment is indicated
  - Closed treatment includes posterior force on the lateral shoulder or clavicle with a sand bag placed between the scapulae
  - Open reduction is indicated if the patient is symptomatic or if irreducible dislocation is present
  - Never use pins or wires due to risk of migration into the mediastinum

- **Pearl**

Because the medial epiphysis of the clavicle does not completely fuse until 24 y, physeal injury can occur before this age.

References

Bicos J, Nicholson GP: Treatment and results of sternoclavicular joint injuries. Clin Sports Med 2003;22:359. [PMID: 12825536]

Wettstein M, et al.: Anterior subluxation after reduction of a posterior traumatic sterno-clavicular dislocation: a case report and a review of the literature. Knee Surg Sports Traumatol Arthrosc 2004;12:453. [PMID: 15175849]

Bicipital Tendonitis

ICD-9: 726.12

- ■ Essentials of Diagnosis
  - Probably caused by the same mechanism that causes rotator cuff impingement syndrome (ie, impingement beneath the coracoacromial arch)
  - Pain in the proximal humerus and shoulder joint
  - Tenderness to direct palpation of the tendon with the arm internally rotated 10 degrees
  - Speed test: resisted elevation of the supinated arm with the elbow extended
  - Yergason test: resisted supination with elbow flexed is positive for pain at the bicipital groove

- ■ Differential Diagnosis
  - Rotator cuff tendonitis
  - Rotator cuff tear
  - Biceps tendon rupture
  - Biceps tendon subluxation

- ■ Treatment
  - Treatment focuses on identifying and addressing the cause (eg, shoulder impingement or bicipital tendon subluxation) along with rotator cuff strengthening exercises
  - NSAIDs for pain relief
  - Restriction of activities initially, followed by a slow resumption after a period of rest
  - Strengthening of the muscles that assist the biceps in elbow flexion and forearm supination is beneficial
  - Steroid injections should be made into the sheath of the biceps tendon, not into the substance of the tendon!
  - Surgical release with or without tenodesis may be beneficial in refractory cases

- ■ Pearl

Tendonitis usually occurs secondary to impingement of the tendon on the acromion or tendon subluxation from the proximal humeral groove.

References

Holtby R, Razmiou H: Accuracy of the Speed's and Yergason's tests in detecting biceps pathology and SLAP lesions: comparison with arthroscopic findings. Arthroscopy 2004;20:231. [PMID 15007311]

Patton WC, McCluskey GM 3rd: Biceps tendinitis and subluxation. Clin Sports Med 2001;20:505. [PMID: 11494838]

Biceps Tendon Rupture

ICD-9: 840.8; 727.62 Nontraumatic

■ Essentials of Diagnosis

- Mechanism: forceful flexion of the arm
- Obvious deformity is seen in long head ruptures, with distal migration of the muscle
- Weakness occurring with long head rupture is usually confined to supination activities
- Anterior shoulder pain and tenderness
- Speed test: resisted elevation of the supinated arm with the elbow extended
- Yergason test: resisted supination with the elbow flexed is positive for pain at the bicipital groove
- Distal biceps rupture produces elbow flexion weakness

■ Differential Diagnosis

- Rotator cuff tear
- Bicipital tendonitis
- Bicipital subluxation

■ Treatment

- Long head rupture: tenodesis (in young active patient) or conservative management
- Distal biceps rupture: tendon reconstruction regardless of age

■ Pearl

Rupture of the long head of the biceps tendon is a harbinger of rotator cuff tears in middle-aged and older athletes.

References

Bernstein AD, et al.: Distal biceps tendon ruptures: a historical perspective and current concepts. Am J Orthop 2001;30:193. [PMID: 11300127]

Vidal AF, et al.: Biceps tendon and triceps tendon injuries. Clin Sports Med 2004;23:707. [PMID: 15474231]

Impingement Syndrome

ICD-9: 726.2

- **Essentials of Diagnosis**

  - Can occur with repetitive overhead activities as a result of mechanical impingement of the rotator cuff and humeral head against the acromion
  - The supraspinatus tendon is most susceptible to impingement
  - The weak rotator cuff fails to depress the humeral head, leading to impingement
  - Positive impingement test (passive forward flexion of the internally rotated shoulder causes pain—Neer impingement sign); pain is relieved after the injection of lidocaine into the subacromial bursa
  - Pain with passive internal rotation of the shoulder while the arm is forward-flexed (Hawkins sign)
  - Tenderness localized over the lateral aspect of the acromion
  - Prolonged overhead activity exacerbates symptoms
  - Radiographs show the shape of the acromion in supraspinatus outlook view
  - MRI may reveal cuff changes

- **Differential Diagnosis**

  - Neoplasm in patients with atypical history
  - Cervical radiculitis
  - Joint subluxation
  - Frozen shoulder
  - Acromioclavicular joint arthritis

- **Treatment**

  - Physical therapy for rotator cuff strengthening and range of motion; NSAIDs help provide pain relief while strengthening progresses
  - Acromioplasty is successful in 85% of cases when conservative measures fail

- **Pearl**

Impingement is associated with a hooked (type III) acromion on the supraspinatus outlet view.

References

Ardic F, et al.: Shoulder impingement syndrome: relationships between clinical, functional, and radiologic findings. Am J Phys Med Rehabil 2006;85:53. [PMID: 16357549]

Koester MC, et al.: Shoulder impingement syndrome. Am J Med 2005;188:452. [PMID: 15866244]

Moraq Y, et al.: MR imaging of rotator cuff injury: what the clinician needs to know. Radiographics 2006;26:1045. [PMID: 16844931]

Glenohumeral Joint Instability

ICD-9: 755.59

- ■ Essentials of Diagnosis
  - • Chronic unidirectional or multidirectional instability
  - • TUBS: instability caused by Traumatic event, is Unidirectional, associated with a Bankart lesion, and often requires Surgery
  - • AMBRI: Atraumatic, Multidirectional, may be Bilateral, best treated by Rehabilitation, Inferior capsular shift is the surgery performed if rehabiliation fails
  - • Sulcus sign is suggestive of multidirectional instability (also inferior laxity): with arm at side, distraction force to the humerus causes the shoulder area just below the acromion to hollow out; discomfort occurs if inferior instability is present
  - • Anterior instability: apprehension test is positive when arm is in an externally rotated and abducted position; pressure on the humeral head in the anterior direction causes guarding
  - • Posterior instability: apprehension test is positive when arm is in an internally rotated, flexed, and adducted position; a posterior force causes guarding

- ■ Differential Diagnosis
  - • Multidirectional, anterior, inferior, or posterior instability
  - • SLAP (superior labrum anterior-posterior) lesion

- ■ Treatment
  - • Treatment for instability should begin with a rehabilitation program for the shoulder; rotator cuff and shoulder girdle strengthening is basic to the program
  - • Failure to alleviate instability that interferes with sleep, work, or sports activities suggests the need for surgery, especially in TUBS patients; arthroscopic Bankart repairs and capsular shifts can minimize surgical trauma and speed rehabilitation
  - • Approach multidirectional instability with caution; ensure that all nonoperative measures have been attempted before proceeding to surgery

- ■ Pearl

The majority of glenohumeral dislocations and subluxations are in the anteroinferior direction.

References

Cole BJ, et al.: Arthroscopic treatment of anterior glenohumeral instability: indications and techniques. Instr Course Lect 2004;53:545. [PMID: 15116643]

Millett PJ, et al.: Open operative treatment for anterior shoulder instability: when and why? J Bone Joint Surg Am 2005;87:419. [PMID: 15687170]

Acromioclavicular Joint Arthropathy

ICD-9: 715.11

■ Essentials of Diagnosis

- Osteoarthritis (OA; primarily or secondary to trauma) or osteolysis can develop in the acromioclavicular joint (ACJ)
- Osteolysis typically occurs in young athletes who do strength training or collision sports; the distal end of the clavicle undergoes osteolysis, causing pain at the ACJ
- As with OA of other joints, OA of the ACJ is due to repetitive use and a genetic predisposition
- Physical exam reveals pain with palpation, pain during "crossover" testing (ie, reaching over the body and grabbing the contralateral shoulder with the ipsilateral hand), and pain at the ACJ during glenohumeral extension
- If the source of the pain is unclear, a diagnostic injection of local anesthetic into the ACJ is helpful
- Radiographs show an apparent resorption of the lateral clavicle in osteolysis, and joint space narrowing, osteophyte formation, subchondral cysts, and subchondral sclerosis in OA

■ Differential Diagnosis

- ACJ separation or strain
- Rotator cuff impingement
- Rotator cuff tear
- SLAP (superior labrum anterior-posterior) tear
- Cervical radiculopathy
- Cervical spondylosis

■ Treatment

- Initially treat all patients conservatively with NSAIDs and activity modification
- Steroid injections are frequently helpful in alleviating pain
- If conservative treatment fails, an arthroscopic or open distal clavicle resection (Mumford procedure) often alleviates symptoms
- During the Mumford procedure, 8–10 mm of the lateral clavicle is resected; if less is removed, pain can persist; if more is removed, ACJ instability can develop

■ Pearl

Thirty percent of MRIs in patients with an asymptomatic ACJ demonstrate ACJ arthritis. An asymptomatic ACJ does not require treatment even if the MRI is positive.

Reference

Buttaci CJ, et al.: Osteoarthritis of the acromioclavicular joint: a review of anatomy, biomechanics, diagnosis, and treatment. Am J Phys Med Rehabil 2004;83:791. [PMID: 15385790]

Adhesive Capsulitis (Frozen Shoulder)

ICD-9: 726.0

- **Essentials of Diagnosis**
  - May be traumatic or idiopathic
  - Idiopathic disease is more common in older patients (40–60 y), diabetics, and women; other predisposing factors include cervical, neurologic, cardiac, neoplastic, pulmonary, and personality disorders
  - Natural history has 3 phases: painful freezing phase (2–9 mo); progressive stiffness phase, in which motion becomes stiff in all planes while pain decreases; and resolution phase (1 mo to several years), during which range of motion (ROM) gradually improves
  - Exam shows loss of both active and passive ROM; internal rotation is usually first affected
  - Radiography is not helpful; arthrography reveals markedly decreased joint capsule capacity

- **Differential Diagnosis**
  - Rotator cuff tear
  - Rotator cuff tendonitis

- **Treatment**
  - Progressive ROM with physical therapy is effective
  - Oral steroids are not as effective as intra-articular steroids
  - Arthroscopic capsular release is becoming the accepted treatment for this process and seems to decrease the time required to achieve and maintain motion

- **Pearl**

Manipulation under anesthesia is effective in obtaining increased ROM but is associated with significant iatrogenic intra-articular damage.

References

Loew M, et al.: Intraarticular lesions in primary frozen shoulder after manipulation under general anesthesia. J Shoulder Elbow Surg 2005;14:16. [PMID: 15723009]

Ryans I, et al.: A randomized controlled trial of intra-articular triamcinolone and/or physiotherapy in shoulder capsulitis. Rheumatology (Oxford) 2005;44:529. [PMID: 15657070]

Glenoid Labrum Injury

ICD-9: 831.0

- **Essentials of Diagnosis**
  - Occurs from repetitive shoulder motion or acute trauma (ie, a fall onto an outstretched arm)
  - Anterior subluxation may lead to anteroinferior labral tears
  - Pain interrupts smooth functioning of the shoulder
  - Pain occurs on external rotation with arm abducted; a "pop" or "click" may be felt with forced external rotation
  - Rotator cuff weakness
  - CT or MRI arthrogram is diagnostic

- **Differential Diagnosis**
  - Glenohumeral joint instability
  - Rotator cuff tear
  - Loose body in joint

- **Treatment**
  - Conservative management, consisting of range of motion exercises with gradual return to activities, is often successful
  - Failure of nonoperative treatment is an indication for arthroscopic debridement of the labrum
  - Baseball pitchers may be ready to throw in 3 mo

- **Pearl**

Posterior glenoid labral tears are associated with glenoid dysplasia as evaluated on MRI.

Reference

Guanche CA, Jones DC: Clinical testing for tears of the glenoid labrum. Arthroscopy 2003;19:517. [PMID: 12724682]

SLAP Lesions

ICD-9: 840.7

- Essentials of Diagnosis
  - The acronym SLAP (superior labrum anterior-posterior) describes a superior, anterior-to-posterior glenoid labral degeneration or tear involving the origin of the long head of the biceps
  - There are several types, but type II (detachment of the superior labrum from the glenoid) is the most common
  - Patients present with nonspecific shoulder pain associated with activity, stiffness, and instability
  - To test for SLAP (suggestive, not diagnostic), the arm is extended and adducted across the chest with the forearm pronated; a positive test elicits pain at the bicipital groove, apprehension, or a "click," which is diminished with repetition of the maneuver with the forearm supinated

- Differential Diagnosis
  - Glenoid labral tear
  - Bankart lesion
  - Glenohumeral instability
  - Rotator cuff tear

- Treatment
  - Treatment is either arthroscopic repair of the lesion to the glenoid, when the biceps tendon is not involved, or tenotomy of the biceps tendon with or without tenodesis, if the tendon is involved

- Pearl

SLAP lesions may lead to posterior glenolabral cysts, which can be a cause of suprascapular nerve compression.

Reference

Swaringen JC, et al.: Electromyographic analysis of physical examination tests for type II superior labrum anterior-posterior lesions. J Shoulder Elbow Surg 2006;15:576. [PMID: 16979052]

Calcific Tendonitis of the Rotator Cuff

ICD-9: 726.11

- **Essentials of Diagnosis**
  - An acute or chronic condition of the shoulder in which calcium deposits develop within the rotator cuff tendons
  - The cause of the calcification is unknown
  - Patients are usually >30 y; incidence is higher in females, diabetics, and patients with concurrent rotator cuff tears
  - Symptoms are similar to those of impingement syndrome (ie, night pain, pain with overhead activity)
  - Physical exam reveals tenderness over the greater tuberosity; there often is pain with passive forward flexion (Neer sign), as well as with forward flexion to 90 degrees with subsequent internal rotation (Hawkins sign)
  - Plain radiographs typically show the calcified tendon

- **Differential Diagnosis**
  - Rotator cuff tear
  - Rotator cuff impingement
  - Shoulder instability
  - SLAP (superior labrum anterior-posterior) tear
  - Cervical radiculopathy or spondylosis

- **Treatment**
  - Initial management includes activity modification and NSAIDs
  - Steroids are often helpful in alleviating symptoms but should not be used in patients with concurrent rotator cuff tears
  - Needle lavage has been used to break up the calcification and decrease symptoms, but efficacy is limited
  - Calcification has also been treated with extracorporeal shock wave therapy
  - Surgery is indicated in patients whose symptoms are recalcitrant to conservative treatment; the calcification can be removed arthroscopically or in an open procedure

- **Pearl**

If a rotator cuff tear is not present prior to surgical treatment of a calcific tendonitis, one may exist after removal of a large deposit. In such cases, a repair of the defect in the rotator cuff is necessary.

Reference

Hurt G, Baker CL: Calcific tendonitis of the shoulder. Orthop Clin North Am 2003;34:567. [PMID: 14984196]

Acromioclavicular Separation

ICD-9: 831.04

- **Essentials of Diagnosis**
  - Caused by direct trauma to the acromioclavicular joint (ACJ)
  - Six types: *type I*—isolated strain of ACJ capsule, no displacement; *type II*—disruption of capsule and partial disruption of coracoclavicular (CC) ligaments, <50% vertical displacement of clavicle; *type III*—complete disruption of capsule and CC ligaments, 50–100% displacement; *type IV*—posterior displacement; *type V*—100–300% vertical displacement; *type VI*—inferior displacement
  - Physical exam findings include pain and deformity
  - Radiographic exam is negative for type I; types II, III, V, and VI are readily seen on plain radiographs; in type IV, posterior displacement may be missed on an AP radiograph, and an axial radiograph or CT scan is required

- **Differential Diagnosis**
  - Lateral clavicle fracture
  - Rotator cuff impingement
  - Rotator cuff tear
  - Shoulder instability
  - Scapulothoracic dissociation

- **Treatment**
  - Conservative treatment, types I and II: during the initial 2 wk, provide pain control (sling, NSAIDs, ice) and start range of motion exercises
  - Type III: treatment is controversial; in patients with high demand (ie, throwing athletes), surgical repair is warranted; in others, an attempt at conservative treatment is commonly employed
  - Types IV—VI: surgical repair or reconstruction

- **Pearl**

Type I and II ACJ separations respond well to nonoperative treatment. However, patients with these injuries can develop ACJ arthritis later because the clavicle and acromion remain in contact with each other.

Reference

Mazzocca AD, et al.: Evaluation and treatment of acromioclavicular joint injuries. Am J Sports Med 2007;35:316. [PMID 17251175]

Scapular Winging

ICD-9: 723.4 Brachial neuritis; 719.4 Shoulder pain;
726.10 Disorder of shoulder muscle

- ■ Essentials of Diagnosis
  - Abnormal motion of scapulothoracic articulation that may be primary (from weakness of muscles that control motion of the scapulothoracic articulation) or secondary (from abnormalities of the glenohumeral joint that cause compensatory winging)
  - May have *trapezial (weakness) winging* (eg, from spinal accessory nerve injury), *serratus anterior (weakness) winging* (eg, from long thoracic nerve injury), or *rhomboideus (weakness) winging* (eg, dorsal scapular nerve injury); nerve injuries can be iatrogenic or due to trauma or virus (Parson-Turner syndrome)
  - On physical exam, winging is accentuated when patient pushes against a wall; in trapezial winging, scapula moves downward and tip of scapula rotates laterally; in serratus anterior winging, scapula moves upward and tip of the scapula rotates medially
  - Muscle atrophy; often, loss of abduction and forward flexion
  - EMG/NCS can aid in making the diagnosis

- ■ Differential Diagnosis
  - Fracture malunion
  - Scapulothoracic contracture
  - Osteochondroma of the scapula
  - Voluntary winging
  - Muscle (serratus, trapezium, rhomboid) avulsion or laceration
  - Multidirectional instability (MDI) of the shoulder

- ■ Treatment
  - Etiology determines the treatment: if viral, physical therapy and time will resolve symptoms; nerve repair will resolve traumatic laceration; tumor removal will relieve compression
  - Consider surgery for patients who have persistent disability after 1 y of conservative treatment for iatrogenic causes
  - Surgical treatment options: for trapezial paralysis, levator scapulae and rhomboids can be transferred laterally (Eden-Lange transfer); for serratus anterior paralysis, sternocostal head of the pectoralis major can be transferred to inferior corner of the scapula (Marmor-Bechtol transfer); an alternative is scapulothoracic fusion

- ■ Pearl

Rarely, voluntary muscle forces can cause scapular winging. Voluntary winging often has a psychological component.

Reference

Kuhn JE, et al.: Scapular winging. J Amer Acad Orthop Surg 1995;3:319. [PMID: 10790670]

Rotator Cuff Tear

ICD-9: 840.4

■ Essentials of Diagnosis

- Tear at the tendinous insertion of one of the rotator cuff muscles (supraspinatus, infraspinatus, subscapularis, teres minor); most often the supraspinatus tendon is torn
- Associated with repetitive overhead activity, biceps tendon ruptures, and advanced age
- Uncommon before 40 y unless associated with high-energy trauma
- After a shoulder dislocation in patients older than 60 y, there is 60% chance of concurrent rotator cuff tear
- Patient has significant weakness and pain in abduction and external rotation
- Large tears can progress to humeral head elevation, articulation of the humeral head with the acromial, and significant glenohumeral arthritis (ie, rotator cuff arthropathy)
- Diagnosed radiographically by MRI

■ Differential Diagnosis

- Rotator cuff impingement
- Acromioclavicular joint arthritis
- Glenohumeral arthritis
- Shoulder instability
- Cervical strain or cervical radiculopathy

■ Treatment

- If tear is a partial or small, a trial of conservative treatments is warranted; conservative treatment includes NSAIDs, along with physical therapy to strengthen the rotator cuff and scapular stabilizer muscles
- Steroid injections are contraindicated because they can cause the remaining cuff to weaken and tear further
- Surgical treatment is direct repair of the rotator cuff back to its bony insertion on the greater tuberosity; surgery can be open, mini open (small split in the deltoid), or arthroscopic

■ Pearl

Patients often complain of shoulder pain at night that prevents them from going to sleep or wakes them from sleep.

Reference

Oh LS, Wolf BR, Hall MP, et al.: Indications for rotator cuff repair: a systematic review. Clin Orthop 2007;455:52. [PMID: 17179786]

Shoulder Injuries in the Throwing Athlete

ICD-9: not applicable

- **Essentials of Diagnosis**
  - Throwing athletes (baseball, football, javelin) generate tremendous force to throw at high speeds; the shoulder helps generate this force and is therefore susceptible to injury
  - Baseball pitchers adaptively increase external rotation (ER) and decrease internal rotation (IR) in their throwing shoulder
  - The throwing shoulder can develop internal impingement (eg, posterior rotator cuff impinges against posterior glenoid), SLAP tears (eg, superior labrum and biceps anchor detach from superior labrum), anterior instability, scapular winging or dyskinesis, or posterior capsular tears (Bennett lesions)
  - Physical exam: positive apprehension test causing pain; relocation test that relieves pain; increased ER and decreased IR in affected shoulder compared with contralateral side
  - Plain radiographs are often normal; posterior capsular avulsion can sometimes be seen
  - Obtain an MRI or MRI arthrogram if a labral tear is suspected (most sensitive imaging study); if posterior impingement is a concern, obtain ABER (arm in abduction and ER) view

- **Differential Diagnosis**
  - SLAP (superior labrum anterior-posterior) tear
  - Rotator cuff tear
  - Rotator cuff or biceps tendonitis
  - Acromioclavicular joint arthritis
  - Unstable os acromiale

- **Treatment**
  - Physical therapy (mainstay of treatment): rotator cuff and scapular stabilizer strengthening; stretching the posterior capsule is important; careful evaluation of form is also beneficial to prevent recurrence
  - If conservative treatment fails, arthroscopic or open repair is warranted; damaged structures will have to be repaired (SLAP, rotator cuff, labrum); sometimes the stretched anterior capsule needs to be tightened and the tight posterior capsule needs to be released

- **Pearl**

Often the cause of a shoulder problem in the throwing athlete is weakness or imbalance of the legs or torso.

Reference

Burkhart SS, et al.: The disabled throwing shoulder: spectrum of pathology. Part I: pathoanatomy and biomechanics. Arthroscopy 2003;19:404. [PMID: 12671624]

Medial Epicondylitis (Golf Elbow)

ICD-9: 726.31

- **Essentials of Diagnosis**
  - Caused by tendinopathy at the attachment of the flexor muscles at their origin
  - Pain occurs along the medial elbow and worsens on resisted forearm pronation or wrist flexion; tenderness is ~5 mm distal and anterior to the midpoint of the medial epicondyle
  - Ulnar nerve compression syndrome is present in a high percentage of patients treated surgically
  - Radiographs are not typically helpful, except to rule out other cause of medial elbow pain

- **Differential Diagnosis**
  - Medial collateral ligament disruption
  - Osteochondral lesions of the trochlea and olecranon
  - Medial compartment elbow arthritis
  - Ulnar neurapraxia (cubital tunnel syndrome)

- **Treatment**
  - Treatment modalities include bracing physical therapy, rest, ice, and injections of steroid for tendinopathy; medial epicondylitis treated with steroid injections has a high rate of recurrence after good early results
  - Physical therapy for flexion contracture
  - Surgical debridement may be helpful in recalcitrant cases, but the tendon should not be released or should be reattached, if released

- **Pearl**

Physical therapy and NSAIDs are successful in >90% of patients with tendinopathy, but the epicondylitis may not resolve for 1 y.

References

Ciccotti MC, et al.: Diagnosis and treatment of medial epicondylitis of the elbow. Clin Sports Med 2004;23:693. [PMID: 15474230]

Hume PA, et al.: Epicondylar injury in sport: epidemiology, type, mechanism, assessment, management and prevention. Sports Med 2006;36:151. [PMID: 16464123]

Pienimaki TT, et al.: Chronic medial and lateral epicondylitis: a comparison of pain, disability, and function. Arch Phys Med Rehabil 2002;83:317. [PMID: 11887110]

Lateral Epicondylitis (Tennis Elbow)

ICD-9: 726.32

- **Essentials of Diagnosis**
    - Caused by tendinopathy at the attachment of the extensor muscles at their origin
    - Repetitive wrist extension puts patients at risk
    - Symptoms are usually more bothersome than disabling
    - Pain occurs with resisted supination and wrist extension with elbow extended
    - Tenderness is localized over the origin of the extensor carpi radialis brevis (ECRB)
    - Radiographs occasionally show soft tissue calcification at the origin of the ECRB; radiographs also rule out other diagnoses

- **Differential Diagnosis**
    - Radiocapitellar arthritis
    - Posterior interosseous nerve compression
    - Osteochondritis dissecans of the capitellum

- **Treatment**
    - Conservative treatment is directed at decreasing specific activities that cause pain; use of a tennis elbow band helps to diminish symptoms; patients should have tennis lessons to learn correct use of a racquet; wrist extension strengthening exercises should be included
    - NSAIDs can be helpful in treating symptoms, as can a steroid injection into the point of maximum tenderness
    - Surgery is indicated in recalcitrant cases; several approaches are helpful but all include release of the common extensor tendon

- **Pearl**

Corticosteroid injections have good results initially but high recurrence rates after 6 wk.

References

Bisset L, et al.: Mobilisation with movement and exercise, corticosteroid injection, or wait and see for tennis elbow: randomized trial. BMJ 2006;333:939. [PMID: 17012266]

Kim DH, et al.: Surgical treatment and outcomes in 45 cases of posterior interosseous nerve entrapments and injuries. J Neurosurg 2006;104:766. [PMID: 16703882]

Pienimaki TT, et al.: Chronic medial and lateral epicondylitis: a comparison of pain, disability, and function. Arch Phys Med Rehabil 2002;83:317. [PMID: 11887110]

Throwing Injuries in the Pediatric Elbow

ICD-9: not applicable

- Essentials of Diagnosis
  - The elbow undergoes large valgus forces (64 N-m) in throwing sports; the medial side can have tension injuries—medial apophysitis, medial epicondyle avulsions, flexor tendonitis, ulnar nerve neuritis, or medial collateral (MCL) injuries; the lateral side can have compression injuries—osteochondritis of the capitellum (little leaguer's elbow) or osteochondrosis of the capitellum epiphysis (Panner disease)
  - Medial apophysitis affects adolescents 14–17 y, occurs just before physis closure, and can lead to fracture through medial physeal avulsion; little leaguer's elbow affects children 11–14 y and is non-reversible; Panner disease affects children 7–10 y and is reversible
  - History of gradually increasing pain during throwing and decreased throwing velocity; sometimes a sudden "pop" is felt
  - Physical exam reveals tenderness over the affected area, swelling, and decreased range of motion
  - Plain radiographs can reveal avulsion injuries and advanced osteochondritis or osteochondrosis; MRI reveals osteochondritis or osteochondrosis; MRI arthrogram is best for diagnosing ligament tears

- Differential Diagnosis
  - Osteochondritis of the capitellum (little leaguer's elbow)
  - Osteochondrosis of the capitellum (Panner disease)
  - Medial apophysitis or avulsion of medial epiphysis
  - Loose body

- Treatment
  - Medial epiphyseal avulsions typically require surgery if displaced >5 mm; treat osteochondritis and osteochondrosis with rest and splinting in severe cases; cessation of throwing activity for varying amount of time is necessary; Panner disease usually resolves and child can return to throwing sports
  - Osteochondrosis is an ominous sign and necessitates that the child stops all sports requiring high-velocity throwing

- Pearl

To prevent little leaguer's elbow, the American Little League limits pitchers to 200 pitches per week.

Reference

Kobayashi K, et al.: Lateral compression injuries in the pediatric elbow: Panner's disease and osteochondritis dissecans of the capitellum. J Am Acad Orthop Surg 2004;12:246. [PMID: 15473676]

Elbow Injuries in the Throwing Athlete

ICD-9: not applicable

- ■ Essentials of Diagnosis
  - Throwing athletes place tremendous stress on the elbow joint to achieve high throwing speeds; valgus forces at the elbow during throwing can produce tension lesions on the medial (ulnar) elbow
  - Common pathologic injuries include medial ulnar collateral ligament (MUCL) strain, stretch, or tear; valgus extension overload (VEO) of the olecranon against the medial olecranon fossa; medial epicondylitis; flexor tendonitis; and ulnar nerve neuritis
  - Physical exam often reveals pain or laxity during valgus exam of the elbow
  - Flexion contracture of the elbow is frequently present
  - In VEO, pain is most pronounced if the elbow is rapidly brought to full extension
  - Radiographs may show avulsion injuries of the ligaments or osteophytes on the medial olecranon; MRI arthrogram shows a "t" sign if the MUCL is completely disrupted

- ■ Differential Diagnosis
  - Etiologies mentioned above
  - Osteoarthritis of the elbow
  - Loose body

- ■ Treatment
  - Initially treat valgus overload injuries conservatively for 12 wk with activity modification and physical therapy modalities (ice, iontophoresis, etc)
  - During rehabilitation, examine the throwing mechanics as a whole; elbow problems often develop because of lower extremity or torso weakness during throwing
  - If conservative treatment fails, surgical correction is warranted; the MUCL can be reconstructed ("Tommy John's" procedure); VEO impingement can be arthroscopically debrided

- ■ Pearl

Examination of valgus laxity of the elbow is difficult because the humerus and scapula can externally and internally rotate. To prevent scapular and humeral rotation during the exam, have the patient lie supine on a firm table to lock the scapula. Maximally rotate the humerus externally. Then test the elbow in valgus stress with the elbow at 30 degrees.

Reference

Cain EL, et al.: Elbow injuries in the throwing athlete. Am J Sports Med 2003;31:621. [PMID: 12860556]

Pes Anserinus Bursitis

ICD-9: 726.61

- Essentials of Diagnosis
  - The pes anserinus bursa is located between the sartorius, gracilis, and semitendinosus tendons and the superficial medial collateral ligament
  - Pes anserinus bursitis occurs rarely and is overdiagnosed
  - Repetitive flexion and extension can inflame the bursa
  - The area is point tender and occasionally boggy and edematous
  - Radiographs are negative and ultrasound, positive

- Differential Diagnosis
  - Medial meniscus tear
  - Medial tibial plateau fracture or bone bruise
  - Medial collateral ligament bursitis

- Treatment
  - Steroid injection at the site of maximum tenderness is helpful
  - Avoidance of activities that cause the pain, along with ice and NSAIDs, is indicated

- Pearl

Tenderness of the medial tibial plateau (pes anserinus area) is not likely to be pes anserinus bursitis unless proven on ultrasound.

References

Uson J, et al.: Pes anserinus tendino-bursitis: what are we talking about? Scand J Rheumatol 2000;29:184. [PMID: 10898072]

Yoon HS, et al.: Correlation between ultrasonographic findings and the response to corticosteroid injection in pes anserinus tendinobursitis syndrome in knee osteoarthritis patients. J Korean Med Sci 2005;20:109. [PMID: 15716614]

Bone Bruises

ICD-9: 733.90

- ■ Essentials of Diagnosis
  - Also called *post-traumatic occult bone lesions*
  - Radiologic definition: subcortical area of signal loss (various shapes) on T_1-weighted images and of increased signal intensity on T_2-weighted and FIR images
  - Often found in the femur or tibia at the knee
  - Tender to palpation
  - Radiographs are negative for fracture
  - MRI of patients with acute ACL tears will often show bone bruising of the middle of the lateral femoral condyle and the posterior of the lateral tibial plateau

- ■ Differential Diagnosis
  - Meniscal tear
  - Early degenerative joint disease
  - Plica syndrome
  - Pes anserinus bursitis

- ■ Treatment
  - Bone bruises probably exist on a continuum between fracture and normal, where swelling occurs in the bone from trauma
  - Treat symptomatically, with activity modification and orthoses to unload the joint
  - Prognosis is generally good; a 50% reduction in bruise volume is seen on scanning in 80% of patients at 12–14 wk

- ■ Pearl

A high incidence of injury to other joint structures is associated with bone bruises.

References

Boks SS, et al.: Follow-up of occult bone lesions detected at MR imaging: a systematic review. Radiology 2006;238:853. [PMID: 16452394]

Davies NH, et al.: Magnetic resonance imaging of bone bruising in the acutely injured knee—short-term outcome. Clin Radiol 2004;59:439. [PMID: 15081849]

Patellofemoral Arthralgia

ICD-9: 717.7

- ■ Essentials of Diagnosis
  - Pain going up or down stairs or hills; instability with activities
  - No history of trauma; swelling is uncommon
  - More common in female than in male patients
  - Physical exam may show valgus alignment of the knees, femoral anteversion (increased internal rotation compared with external rotation), quadriceps weakness, and generalized laxity of ligaments
  - No effusion; ligament exam is normal and symmetric
  - Obtain radiographs of the knee (sunrise or Merchant view is essential) and possibly hip; knee radiographs may show slight subluxation of the patellae

- ■ Differential Diagnosis
  - Patellofemoral arthritis, subluxation, or instability
  - Plica syndrome
  - Osgood-Schlatter disease
  - Chondromalacia patella
  - Jumper's knee
  - Osteochondritis dissecans
  - Hip disorders

- ■ Treatment
  - Ice, rest, and NSAIDs for acute pain are indicated, along with quadriceps strengthening and hamstring stretching
  - Patellar stabilizing brace may be helpful

- ■ Pearl

Hip disorders should be considered as a cause of knee pain complaints in children.

References

Dye SF: The pathophysiology of patellofemoral pain: a tissue homeostasis perspective. Clin Orthop 2005;436:100. [PMID: 15995427]

Post WR: Anterior knee pain: diagnosis and treatment. Am Acad Orthop Surg 2005;13:534. [PMID: 16330515]

Meniscal Injury

ICD-9: 836.1 Lateral; 836.0 Medial

■ Essentials of Diagnosis

- Medial tears are more common than lateral; peak incidence in third and fourth decades; after age 50, tears are more commonly due to arthritis than trauma
- Caused by axial loading with rotation, but may be a trivial incident
- Lateral tears may be associated with anterior cruciate ligament (ACL) tears and major sports injuries
- Patients may complain of pain at the joint line area, locking, clicking, giving way, and swelling with activity
- Swelling (effusion) in the joint and joint line tenderness to palpation
- Obtain radiographs to rule out extra-articular causes of knee pain; MRI or arthroscopy confirms the diagnosis

■ Differential Diagnosis

- Early degenerative joint disease
- Post-traumatic occult bone lesion (bone bruise)
- Plica syndrome
- Pes anserinus bursitis

■ Treatment

- Some small tears in the peripheral portion of the meniscus will heal; larger tears require removal of the torn portion (partial meniscectomy) or repair of the torn portion
- Repair may be attempted in patients <40 y; the lack of blood supply to the meniscus more than 4–5 mm from the periphery means that special measures must be taken to promote healing; repair is successful in 50% of knees without ACL tears
- Meniscal transplantation can be attempted and may be of value as lack of a meniscus predisposes to arthrosis

■ Pearl

In patients >40 y, obtain a standing PA Rosenberg view radiograph prior to an MRI for suspicion of a meniscal tear to rule out degenerative arthrosis.

References

Noyes FR, Barber-Westin SD: Meniscus transplantation: indications, techniques, clinical outcomes. Instr Course Lect 2005;54:341. [PMID: 15948463]

Wu WH, et al.: Effects of meniscal and articular surface status on knee stability, function, and symptoms after anterior cruciate ligament reconstruction: a long-term prospective study. Am J Sports Med 2002;30:845. [PMID: 12435651]

Popliteal (Baker) Cyst

ICD-9: 727.51 Baker cyst; 836.0 Meniscal tear;
717.9 Internal derangement of knee

- Essentials of Diagnosis
  - A fluid-filled cyst that occurs between the medial head of the gastrocnemius and semimembranosus tendons; found (less often) on the posterolateral aspect of the knee
  - Cysts are typically filled with a viscous, fibrin-rich fluid and lined with flattened mesothelium-like cells
  - Patients often report a mass and pain in the posterior aspect of the knee; the mass tends to enlarge after vigorous exercise and subside during rest
  - Ultrasound or MRI can identify the cyst; MRI is more frequently used because it is also helpful in identifying concurrent intra-articular pathology
  - Cysts are frequently associated with intra-articular pathology (ie, meniscal tears, degenerative arthritis, or rheumatoid arthritis); 82% of popliteal cysts are associated with meniscal tears (two-thirds, medial meniscus tears; one-third, lateral)

- Differential Diagnosis
  - Benign soft-tissue tumors (lipoma, fibroma, osteochondroma)
  - Malignant lesions in the popliteal fossa (rare; fibrosarcoma or malignant fibrohistiocytoma)
  - Synovitis caused by inflammatory arthritides
  - Meniscal cyst

- Treatment
  - Most adults can be successfully treated nonsurgically
  - Nonsurgical treatment options include NSAIDs and compression sleeves; some authorities advocate aspiration and intracyst injections with corticosteroid
  - If conservative treatment fails and symptoms persist, consider surgical treatment; if intra-articular pathology is present, arthroscopic evaluation and treatment will often alleviate symptoms and decompress the cyst
  - If the cyst is not associated with intra-articular pathology, consider open excision

- Pearl

Popliteal cysts in pediatric patients are typically self-limited, not associated with intra-articular pathology, and should be treated conservatively.

Reference

Fritschy D, et al.: The popliteal cyst. Knee Surg Sports Traumatol Arthrosc 2006;14:623. [PMID 16362357]

Lateral Collateral Ligament (LCL) Injury

ICD-9: 844.0 Acute; 717.81 Chronic

- ■ Essentials of Diagnosis
  - Isolated LCL tear results from direct varus stress to knee at or near full extension; isolated injuries are rare
  - No effusion in isolated injuries; pain is present laterally
  - Three grades of injury (I–III), based on opening of the knee to varus stress at 30 degrees of flexion; grade III is complete
  - Varus knees have more problems with late instability than valgus knees and may experience a lateral "thrust" in stance phase
  - Varus laxity at 30 degrees of flexion indicates an isolated injury; varus laxity at 0 degrees indicates a more extensive injury
  - Average laxity at 30 degrees of flexion is 7 degrees of opening
  - Obtain radiographs to rule out other pathology; MRI can confirm the diagnosis

- ■ Differential Diagnosis
  - Anterior cruciate ligament (ACL) tear
  - Lateral meniscus tear
  - Osteochondral fracture
  - Lateral compartment degenerative joint disease

- ■ Treatment
  - Treat isolated LCL tears nonoperatively; the goal is to protect the ligament during healing and obtain motion of the knee
  - Treat complete tears surgically; an LCL ligament injury combined with other posterolateral ligament injuries generally fares better with surgical repair in the acute setting
  - Chronic injuries to the posterolateral corner of the knee require reconstruction when symptomatic

- ■ Pearl

Isolated LCL tears are rare and if lateral laxity is seen, posterior or anterior cruciate ligament injuries should be suspected.

Reference

Fanelli GC: Surgical treatment of lateral posterolateral instability of the knee using biceps tendon procedures. Sports Med Arthrosc 2006;14:37. [PMID: 17135944]

Medial Collateral Ligament (MCL) Injury

ICD-9: 844.1 Acute; 717.82 Chronic

- Essentials of Diagnosis
  - Caused by direct valgus stress to the knee or noncontact rotational injury
  - Three grades of injury, based on opening of the knee to valgus stress at 30 degrees of flexion: *grade I* is 1–4 mm, *grade II* is 5–9 mm, and *grade III* is 10–15 mm; grades I and II have an end point whereas grade III has a soft end point to stress
  - Sensation of a "pop" and pain along the course of the MCL is common; immediate swelling is more likely to be an anterior cruciate ligament (ACL) tear or fracture
  - Grade III injuries are often less painful than lower grades
  - Obtain radiographs to rule out other pathology; MRI can confirm the diagnosis

- Differential Diagnosis
  - ACL tear
  - Medial meniscus tear
  - Osteochondral fracture
  - Patellofemoral dislocation

- Treatment
  - Treat isolated MCL tears nonoperatively; the goal is to protect the ligament during healing and obtain motion of the knee
  - Grade III ligament injury combined with other ligament injuries generally fares better with surgical repair

- Pearl

Edema seen on MRI around the MCL after injury is not specific to MCL injuries. It can also be seen with medial and lateral meniscal tears, femoral and tibial chondromalacia, and osteoarthritis.

References

Azar FM: Evaluation and treatment of chronic medial collateral ligament injuries of the knee. Sports Med Arthrosc 2006;14:84. [PMID: 17135952]

Blankenbaker DG, et al.: Is intra-articular pathology associated with MCL edema on MR imaging of the non-traumatic knee? Skeletal Radiol 2005;34:462. [PMID: 15940487]

Anterior Cruciate Ligament (ACL) Tear

ICD-9: 844.2 Acute; 717.83 Chronic

- **Essentials of Diagnosis**
  - Can occur without contact; also by valgus or hyperextension force to knee
  - History of a "pop" at the time of injury and immediate (ie, few hours) swelling and effusion at the knee
  - Patients complain of the knee "giving out" during twisting
  - Physical exam shows a positive anterior drawer sign at 30 degrees (Lachman test) and at 90 degrees; the pivot shift test is also positive
  - Laxity is compared with the other knee, and graded 1–3: grade 1 is 1–5 mm, *grade* 2 is 6–10 mm, and *grade* 3 is >10 mm more than the other knee
  - Obtain radiographs to rule out fracture (eg, Segond fracture)

- **Differential Diagnosis**
  - Chronic ACL tear
  - Avulsion of the tibial insertion in adolescents
  - Multiligamentous injury to the knee

- **Treatment**
  - Conservative management is indicated in patients who can accept modification of activities that produce instability; instability is thought to put the menisci at risk of damage
  - Surgical repair is not successful; reconstruction is an individual decision based on the patient's desires and requirements
  - Patients engaging in competitive athletics generally require reconstruction; the methods vary but generally use autograft to replace the ACL

- **Pearl**

It is important to do the "sag" (Godfrey) test for posterior cruciate ligament laxity. An anterior drawer sign that appears positive actually may reflect the tibia coming from a posterior position to a reduced position, due to PCL laxity.

Reference

Herrington L, et al.: Anterior cruciate ligament reconstruction, hamstring versus bone-patella tendon-bone grafts: a systematic literature review of the outcome from surgery. Knee 2005;12:41. [PMID: 15664877]

Posterior Cruciate Ligament (PCL) Tear

ICD-9: 844.2 Acute; 717.84 Chronic

- ■ Essentials of Diagnosis
  - Occurs from dashboard injury to the tibia or a fall on a flexed knee
  - History of pain and some subjective instability; acute injuries to the PCL can be missed
  - Physical exam shows a positive "sag" (Godfrey) test and a positive posterior drawer sign at 90 degrees (>10 mm, compared with the opposite knee)
  - Obtain radiographs to rule out fracture; posterior subluxation of the tibia on the femur may indicate PCL injury
  - MRI is diagnostic for PCL tear

- ■ Differential Diagnosis
  - Posterolateral corner injuries
  - PCL avulsion fracture
  - Knee dislocation
  - Multiligamentous injury to knee

- ■ Treatment
  - Conservative management is indicated in many patients because the PCL is extra-articular and partial injuries may heal with a good prognosis
  - For complete tears, the knee is immobilized in extension and exercises are started; orthoses are not generally effective in controlling PCL laxity
  - Most surgeons still treat PCL injuries without surgery, but treatment is controversial
  - Surgical reconstruction (indicated for grade III injuries unresponsive to adequate physical therapy) uses autograft or allograft to reconstruct the ligament

- ■ Pearl

Because PCL tears are less common than ACL tears and more difficult to diagnose in the acute setting, a high index of suspicion must be maintained to ensure diagnosis of these injuries.

References

Allen CR, et al.: Posterior cruciate ligament injuries. Curr Opin Rheumatol 2002;14:142. [PMID: 11845019]

Petrigliano FA, McAllister DR: Isolated posterior cruciate ligament injuries of the knee. Sports Med Arthrosc 2006;14:206. [PMID 17135970]

Iliotibial Band (Friction) Syndrome

ICD-9: 726.60

- **Essentials of Diagnosis**
  - Common tendinous overuse syndrome of the knee; the most common cause of lateral knee pain in runners
  - Aggravated by running or cycling; in these activities the iliotibial (I-T) band rubs over the lateral femoral epicondyle repetitively
  - Pain occurs on the lateral side of the knee and is produced with active flexion and extension; grating may be heard
  - Noble test: pain is produced with digital pressure on the lateral epicondyle at 30 degrees when the supine patient extends the knee from the flexed position
  - Radiographs are negative

- **Differential Diagnosis**
  - Lateral meniscus tear
  - Lateral compartment degenerative joint disease
  - Popliteal tenosynovitis

- **Treatment**
  - Treatment should begin with steps to decrease inflammation: activity modification and NSAIDs; in severe cases, corticosteroid injections may be necessary; stretching exercises for the I-T band and hamstrings are beneficial
  - If conservative measures are not sufficient, release of the posterior portion of the I-T band may be necessary

- **Pearl**

The pain occurs at or very near foot contact (~20 degrees of knee flexion) during running and is worsened by downhill running. Sprinting and fast running are less problematic because footstrike occurs at more than 30 degrees of flexion in these activities.

References

Fredericson M, Wolf C: Iliotibial band syndrome in runners: innovations in treatment. Sports Med 2005;35:451. [PMID: 15896092]

Gunter P, Schwellnus MP: Local corticosteroid injection in iliotibial band friction syndrome in runners: a randomised controlled trial. Br J Sports Med 2004;38:269. [PMID: 15155424]

Jumper's Knee (Patellar Tendinopathy)

ICD-9: 726.64

- **Essentials of Diagnosis**
  - Described as a tendonitis or tendinopathy, but histologically a degenerative tendinosis of the knee
  - Common in volleyball players; caused by eccentric overloading
  - Pain occurs along the patellar tendon and the inferior pole of the patella and is elicited when the knee is flexed while actively trying to extend
  - Radiographs are negative, but ultrasound may be helpful in the diagnosis

- **Differential Diagnosis**
  - Patellofemoral arthralgia

- **Treatment**
  - Treatment begins with eccentric quadriceps strengthening exercises and hamstring and quadriceps stretching, although not all studies support the benefits of eccentric training
  - Deep friction massage and ultrasound can be added if needed
  - If an adequate course of exercise does not relieve symptoms, surgical intervention can be considered, but results are supportive of eccentric exercises over surgery

- **Pearl**

Corticosteroid injections are contraindicated due to a high incidence of patellar tendon rupture.

References

Bahr R, et al.: Surgical treatment compared with eccentric training for patellar tendinopathy (Jumper's Knee). A randomized, controlled trial. J Bone Joint Surg Am 2006;88:1689. [PMID: 16882889]

Peers KH, Lysens RJ: Patellar tendinopathy in athletes: current diagnostic and therapeutic recommendations. Sports Med 2005;35:71. [PMID: 15651914].

Turf Toe

ICD-9: 845.12

- ■ Essentials of Diagnosis
  - Sprain of the first metatarsophalangeal (MTP) joint; incidence is increasing due to artificial playing surfaces and lighter athletic footwear
  - Typically caused by hyperextension (85%), but also caused by varus or valgus stress
  - Usually the plantar surface is injured
  - First MTP is painful to motion
  - Radiographs may reveal diastasis of bipartite sesamoids

- ■ Differential Diagnosis
  - Hallus rigidus
  - Spontaneous reduction of first MTD dislocation
  - Gout

- ■ Treatment
  - Protection of the first MTP from motion, especially hyperextension
  - If pain persists despite conservative treatment, repair of the retinaculum and capsule

- ■ Pearl

Range of motion is significantly reduced after turf toe.

Reference

Allen LR, et al.: Turf toe: ligamentous injury of the first metatarsophalangeal joint. Mil Med 2004;169(11):xix–xxiv. [PMID: 15605946]

3

Spinal Problems

Complete Spinal Cord Injury

ICD-9: 806.0x Cervical; 806.2x Thoracic; 806.4x Lumbar; 806.6x Sacral

- Essentials of Diagnosis
  - Total absence of sensation and voluntary motor function caudal to the level of spinal cord injury in the absence of spinal shock
  - Formal diagnosis is established after the period of spinal shock, which typically lasts 24 h
  - Total absence of motor and sensory function below the injury level; the patient is often hyperreflexic
  - No evidence of sacral sparing; presence of the bulbocavernosus reflex
  - Root escape (when some root level function is regained at the level of injury) should not be confused with the return of cord function
  - Careful neurologic exam is necessary to rule out anterior cord or central cord syndromes or other incomplete lesion

- Differential Diagnosis
  - Spinal shock
  - Incomplete lesion

- Treatment
  - Acute management: keep systolic blood pressure >90 mm Hg; restrict fluids for 48 h; keep patient at 100% O_2 saturations
  - If treating within 8 h of injury, give methylprednisolone, 30 mg/kg over 15 min; then, 45 min after bolus, give 5.4 mg/kg/h for 23 h
  - Prevent contractures by splinting immediately, especially elbow and wrist in the upper extremity
  - Aggressive pulmonary hygiene is required
  - Refer for physical and occupational therapy, and psychological counseling

- Pearl

Watch for autonomic dysreflexia (even in acute spinal cord injury) from pain, fecal impaction, and abdominal distention, with blood pressure increasing 35–95% of baseline.

Reference

Krassioukov AV, et al.: Autonomic dysreflexia in acute spinal cord injury: an under-recognized clinical entity. J Neurotrauma 2003;20:707. [PMID: 12965050]

Cervical Strains & Sprains (Whiplash Injury)

ICD-9: 847.0

- ■ Essentials of Diagnosis
  - Pain is the chief complaint
  - Local tenderness; decreased range of motion; headaches, typically occipital; blurred or double vision
  - Dysphagia, hoarseness, jaw pain, difficulty with balance, vertigo
  - Strain refers to muscle injuries; sprain, to ligamentous and capsular injuries
  - Roentgenographic evaluation is indicated

- ■ Differential Diagnosis
  - Fractures
  - Subluxations and dislocations
  - Herniated disk
  - Degenerative disk disease
  - Rheumatoid arthritis
  - Ankylosing spondylitis
  - Infection

- ■ Treatment
  - Initial rest, bed rest if necessary, and soft collar immobilization are indicated, along with use of anti-inflammatory medications
  - Encourage early mobilization with progressive range of motion and weaning from external supports
  - Frequent reassurance is often necessary because symptoms may be long lasting
  - About 42% of patients have persistent symptoms beyond 1 y, with approximately one third having persistent symptoms beyond 2 y; most patients who improve do so within the first 2 mo
  - Factors associated with a poor prognosis include the presence of occipital headaches, interscapular pain, reversal of cervical lordosis, and involvement in litigation or workers' compensation claims; women have a worse prognosis than men

- ■ Pearl

Cervical spine stability must first be verified before the diagnosis of cervical sprain can be made. Examine appropriate C-spine series, including flexion and extension views.

References

Kwon BK, et al.: Subaxial cervical spine trauma. J Am Acad Orthop Surg 2006;14:78. [PMID: 16467183]

Silber JS, et al.: Whiplash: fact or fiction? Am J Orthop 2005;34:23. [PMID: 15707135]

Cervical Radiculopathy

ICD-9: 721.1 Spondylosis; 722.71 Herniated disk

- **Essentials of Diagnosis**
  - Localized disease of the cervical spine related to disk degeneration, with irritation of a particular nerve root
  - Affects 83 in 100,000 adults annually
  - Pain into the dermatomal distributions, below the elbow; often neck pain and referred pain into the shoulder, arm, and interscapular region
  - Tingling or numbness in the nerve root distribution
  - Muscle weakness and reflex changes in the affected root
  - Valsalva and Spurling maneuvers are positive for radicular symptoms
  - *C4–C5 (C5 root)*: numbness—over deltoid; weakness—deltoid, biceps; reflex—biceps; *C5–C6 (C6 root)*: numbness—thumb, index; weakness—biceps; reflex—biceps; *C6–C7 (C7 root)*: numbness—index, middle; weakness—triceps; reflex—triceps; *C7–T1 (C8 root)*: numbness—ring, little; weakness—triceps; reflex—possibly triceps
  - Diagnosis is made clinically and verified by disk space narrowing or herniation on lateral radiograph, MRI, and EMG/NCS

- **Differential Diagnosis**
  - Cervical spondylosis
  - Spinal cord tumor
  - Cardiac pain
  - Peripheral neuropathy
  - Peripheral nerve entrapment

- **Treatment**
  - Depends on symptoms; initial management is soft collar, NSAIDs, and physical therapy; epidural steroids may be helpful; consider surgical intervention if unresponsive to conservative therapy or if neurologic status deteriorates
  - Minimally invasive anterior and posterior techniques for diskectomy are becoming more popular
  - Surgical treatment depends on etiology (eg, diskectomy for herniated disk; decompression and fusion for spondylosis)

- **Pearl**

Cervical radiculopathy is more common in the fourth and fifth decades except at C7–T1 (seventh and eighth decades). The most common site of disk extrusion is C6–C7.

Reference

Aydin Y, et al.: Minimally invasive anterior contralateral approach for the treatment of cervical disc herniation. Surg Neurol 2005;63:210. [PMID: 15734502]

Cervical Spondylosis

ICD-9: 721.0; 721.1 With radiculopathy or myelopathy

- ■ Essentials of Diagnosis
  - Generalized disease of the cervical spine related to disk degeneration; myelopathy, radiculopathy, or both may occur
  - In 90% of men >50 y and women >60 y, radiographs show cervical degeneration: disk changes, then facet arthropathy, and osteophyte formation and ligament instability
  - Patients often present with complaints of shoulder, elbow, wrist, or hand pain and may report headache (if upper cervical spine is affected) and stiff neck
  - Multiple nerve roots may be involved in radicular symptoms, causing arm pain and distal paresthesias
  - Myelopathy may present with radicular symptoms but also loss of balance, broad-based gait, and lower extremity weakness
  - Reflexes are hypoactive in the upper extremity but hyperactive in the lower; possible Babinski reflex and clonus
  - Clinical picture depends on the anatomic level involved
  - On lateral radiographs, the space available for cord (SAC) is measured from the posterior-inferior aspect of the vertebral body to the anterior aspect of the spinous process at the vertebra below; normal SAC is 17 mm; relative stenosis is SAC of 10–13 mm; absolute stenosis is SAC of <10 mm

- ■ Differential Diagnosis
  - Cervical radiculopathy due to cervical disk
  - Spinal cord tumor
  - Rheumatoid arthritis
  - Multiple sclerosis
  - Syringomyelia

- ■ Treatment
  - Depends on symptoms (eg, neck pain alone, radiculopathy, or myelopathy); initial management is soft collar, NSAIDs, and physical therapy; epidural steroids may be helpful
  - Consider surgical intervention if unresponsive to conservative therapy or if neurologic status deteriorates; surgical decompression of cord through an anterior approach allows anterior fusion; cervical disk replacement is probably not appropriate for the generalized disease occurring in spondylosis

- ■ Pearl

Cervical myelopathy is the most common form of spinal cord dysfunction in people older than 55 y.

Reference

Roh JS, et al.: Degenerative disorders of the lumbar and cervical spine. Orthop Clin North Am 2005;36:255. [PMID: 15950685]

Central Cord Syndrome

ICD-9: 806.0x

- ■ Essentials of Diagnosis
  - • Most common incomplete cord lesion; typically occurs after hyperextension injury
  - • Falls are the most common cause, then motor vehicle accidents
  - • Associated with older patients who have preexisting cervical spondylosis
  - • Affects extremities with sacral sparing
  - • Symptoms range from mild to severe
  - • Varying degrees of motor weakness; the upper extremity is affected to a greater degree than the lower extremity
  - • Varying degrees of loss of sensation and bladder function; however, 75% of patients recover some neurologic function
  - • Radiographs may be negative for fracture

- ■ Differential Diagnosis
  - • Anterior cord syndrome
  - • Complete spinal cord injury
  - • Mixed cord syndrome

- ■ Treatment
  - • Most cases are treated conservatively with supportive care
  - • Protect the spine with a cervical orthosis to prevent recurrent hyperextension
  - • Cervical spine decompression may be necessary in select cases

- ■ Pearl

Greater loss of motor function occurs in the upper extremity because there is more gray matter, which is more sensitive to injury due to its higher metabolic rate.

References

Dvorak MF, et al.: Factors predicting motor recovery and functional outcome after traumatic central cord syndrome: a long-term follow-up. Spine 2005;30:2303. [PMID: 16227894]

Song J, et al.: Clinical evaluation of traumatic central cord syndrome: emphasis on clinical significance of prevertebral hyperintensity, cord compression, and intramedullary high-signal intensity on magnetic resonance imaging. Surg Neurol 2006;65:117. [PMID: 16427399]

Song J, et al.: Surgery for acute subaxial traumatic central cord syndrome without fracture or dislocation. J Clin Neurosci 2005;12:438. [PMID: 15925777]

Anterior Cord Syndrome

ICD-9: 806.0x

- ■ Essentials of Diagnosis
  - Immediate paralysis with loss of pain and temperature sensation
  - Preservation of proprioception, vibration, and deep pressure
  - Return of function is seen in approximately 14% of patients
  - Usual patient is a younger (<35 y) trauma victim with a flexion injury
  - Occurs in patients with vertebral body burst fractures and herniated disks that push posterior into anterior cord
  - Also caused by damage to the anterior spinal artery (known as anterior spinal artery syndrome)
  - Radiographs usually define the site of the lesion

- ■ Differential Diagnosis
  - Central cord syndrome
  - Complete spinal cord injury
  - Mixed cord syndromes

- ■ Treatment
  - Most cases are treated conservatively with supportive care unless there is instability of the injured spinal segment or a herniated disk
  - Protect the spine with a cervical orthosis
  - Splinting is necessary to prevent upper and lower extremity flexion contractures

- ■ Pearl

The functional lesion may extend distal to the radiographic lesion because the level of the anterior spinal artery injury is distal.

References

Pollard ME, Apple DF: Factors associated with improved neurological outcomes in patients with incomplete tetraplegia. Spine 2003;28:33. [PMID: 22544952]

Wenger M, et al.: Post-traumatic cervical kyphosis with surgical correction complicated by temporary anterior spinal artery syndrome. J Clin Neurosci 2005;12:193. [PMID: 15749431]

Atlas Fracture (C1 Vertebra)

ICD-9: 806.0 Without spinal cord injury;
806x With spinal cord injury

- **Essentials of Diagnosis**

  - Caused by trauma
  - Vertebral artery injuries may cause basilar insufficiency: vertigo, blurred vision, and nystagmus
  - May be associated with injury to cranial nerves VI–XII and neurapraxia of the suboccipital and greater occipital nerves
  - Patients present with neck pain or a feeling of "instability"
  - Mechanism: axial compression with elements of hyperextension and asymmetric loading of condyles
  - Jefferson fracture is a 4-part fracture of the atlas; most injuries are 2-part and 3-part

- **Differential Diagnosis**

  - Ligamentous injury: transverse ligament rupture, alar ligament rupture
  - Odontoid fracture
  - Hangman's fracture
  - Atlanto-occipital dissociation

- **Treatment**

  - Halo traction or immobilization initially
  - Stable fractures may be treated with rigid cervical orthoses; less stable fractures require prolonged halo vest treatment
  - C1–C2 or occiput to C2 fusion may be necessary for grossly unstable acute fractures or for chronic instability

- **Pearl**

Atlas fractures are rarely associated with neurologic injury but >50% are associated with other cervical spine fractures, especially odontoid.

References

Brolin K: Neck injuries among the elderly in Sweden. Inj Control Saf Promot 2003;10:155. [PMID: 12861914]

Kontautas E, et al.: Management of acute traumatic atlas fractures. J Spinal Disord Tech 2005;18:402. [PMID: 16607070]

Hangman's Fracture

ICD-9: 805.02

- **Essentials of Diagnosis**
  - This is *not* an odontoid fracture; it is a fracture of the ring of C2 producing traumatic spondylolisthesis of C2
  - There is a 30% incidence of concomitant cervical spine fractures
  - Mechanism is hyperextension and axial load
  - Pain, instability, or both are present
  - Patient may have neurologic compromise
  - May be associated with cranial nerve, vertebral artery, or craniofacial injuries
  - Disruption of the C2–C3 disk causes marked instability

- **Differential Diagnosis**
  - Intervertebral disk disruption
  - Ligamentous injury
  - Odontoid fracture
  - Atlas fracture

- **Treatment**
  - Nondisplaced fractures may be treated in a rigid cervical orthosis for 6 wk
  - Unstable injuries require halo traction or immobilization for at least 6 wk
  - Severe disruption may require open treatment with fusion if reduction cannot be maintained

- **Pearl**

Hangman's fracture is one of the few injuries of the cervical spine that can be exacerbated by traction.

References

Li XF, et al.: A systematic review of the management of hangman's fractures. Eur Spine J 2006;15:257. [PMID: 16235100]

Vaccaro AR, et al.: Early halo immobilization of displaced traumatic spondylolisthesis of the axis. Spine 2002;27:2229. [PMID: 12394899]

Fractures of the Lower Cervical Spine

ICD-9: 805.0

- **Essentials of Diagnosis**
  - History of trauma to the neck or head
  - Pain (especially with range of motion)
  - Localized tenderness
  - Careful neurologic exam is important, including sphincter tone and Babinski reflex; findings in anterior cord and central cord lesions may be subtle
  - Diagnosis usually is confirmed with radiographic evaluation
  - CT or MRI may be necessary, if occult
  - Because noncontiguous injury of the spine occurs in ~12% of cases, evaluation of the thoracic and lumbar spine is important

- **Differential Diagnosis**
  - Ligamentous injury (whiplash)
  - Facet joint injury
  - Arthritis or stenosis
  - Disk herniation
  - Infection (tuberculosis)
  - Referred pain (cardiac, etc)
  - Metastases and neoplasms

- **Treatment**
  - Hard collar; spine precautions
  - Surgery for unstable fracture-dislocations to stabilize the spine, prevent progression of neurologic damage, and enable earlier rehabilitation

- **Pearl**

Maintain a high index of suspicion for fracture after a neck injury in patients with ankylosing spondylitis.

Reference

Kwon BK, et al.: Subaxial cervical spine trauma. J Am Acad Orthop Surg 2006;14:78. [PMID: 16467183]

Osteoporotic Vertebral Compression Fracture

ICD-9: 805.2 Thoracic; 805.4 Lumbar

- **Essentials of Diagnosis**
  - Axial pain localized to the fractured level (usually thoracic)
  - Can occur with trivial trauma
  - Incidence is higher in women, Caucasians, Asians, and men >80 y
  - Patients often feel better in a few weeks, only to have an exacerbation of pain from further fracture displacement
  - Tenderness to percussion is localized midline
  - Rule out neurologic injury
  - Plain films usually will make the diagnosis of compression fracture; age of fracture may be difficult to determine
  - Bone scan may be needed occasionally to rule in acute fracture; a bone density scan (DEXA scan) can identify patients at risk

- **Differential Diagnosis**
  - Burst fracture
  - Pathologic fracture from metastasis
  - Myeloma

- **Treatment**
  - Pain management and a thoracolumbar orthosis (usually poorly tolerated)
  - Patients with unstable fractures (>50% loss of height, >30 degrees of kyphosis) or neurologic compromise may need surgical stabilization with anterior decompression and fusion
  - Surgical stabilization of the typical compression fracture can be accomplished by kyphoplasty or vertebroplasty with immediate alleviation of pain

- **Pearl**

Early kyphoplasty (~ first 3 wk) may permit correction of the kyphotic deformity.

Reference

Hulme PA, et al.: Vertebroplasty and kyphoplasty: a systematic review of 69 clinical studies. Spine 2006;31:1983. [PMID: 16924218]

Kyphosis

ICD-9: 737.10

- **Essentials of Diagnosis**
  - Flexion deformity of the spine
  - Normal thoracic kyphosis has a Cobb angle (the angle between lines drawn perpendicular to the endplates of the most cephalad and most caudal vertebra of the curve on the lateral radiograph) that ranges from 25 to 45 degrees
  - Increased kyphosis can be congenital, or a result of trauma or progressive deformity secondary to osteoporosis
  - Scheuermann kyphosis refers to 3 or more wedged vertebral bodies with endplate abnormalities and kyphosis
  - Congenital kyphosis results from failure of vertebral body formation or segmentation

- **Differential Diagnosis**
  - Congenital kyphosis
  - Scheuermann kyphosis
  - Traumatic injury
  - Osteoporotic compression fractures

- **Treatment**
  - Bracing is indicated if kyphosis is >45–55 degrees in a skeletally immature patient
  - Surgery is indicated if kyphosis increases despite bracing in a growing patient, or the Cobb angle is >70 degrees, or both

- **Pearl**

Orthotic treatment of adolescent kyphosis can obtain correction and maintain correction after skeletal maturity.

Reference

Lee SS, et al.: Comparison of Scheuermann kyphosis correction by posterior-only thoracic pedicle screw fixation verus combined anterior/posterior fusion. Spine 2006;31:2316. [PMID: 16985459]

Idiopathic Scoliosis in Adults

ICD-9: 737.30

- **Essentials of Diagnosis**
  - Defined as a lateral deviation and rotation deformity of the spine without an identifiable cause
  - Three categories: infantile, juvenile, and adolescent; all can present in adulthood
  - Right thoracic curves are more common, followed by double major (right thoracic and left lumbar) curves
  - Physical findings include shoulder elevation, waistline asymmetry, rib rotational deformity (rib hump), trunk shift, and limb-length inequality
  - In adults, spinal deformity is usually structural
  - Neurologic exam is usually normal
  - Diagnosis is made with standing AP radiographs of the entire spine

- **Differential Diagnosis**
  - Hormonal disorder
  - Congenital scoliosis
  - Brain stem dysfunction
  - Proprioception disorder
  - Neuromuscular scoliosis
  - Spinal cord abnormalities in patients with neurologic symptoms or left thoracic curves

- **Treatment**
  - In adults, observation and possible surgical intervention are the mainstays of treatment; bracing has no significant role because there is no growth potential
  - Surgical intervention is considered in adults with curves >40–50 degrees, because these patients are at risk for progression, as well as in those with documented progression of >5 degrees; pseudarthrosis after fusion is high (24%)

- **Pearl**

Bracing will not reduce the magnitude of the deformity.

References

Kim YJ, et al.: Pseudarthrosis in long adult spinal deformity instrumentation and fusion to the sacrum: prevalence and risk factor analysis of 144 cases. Spine 2006;31:2329. [PMID: 16985461]

Rinella A, et al.: Late complications of adult idiopathic scoliosis primary fusion to L4 and above: the effect of age and distal fusion level. Spine 2004;29:318. [PMID: 14752356]

Thoracolumbar Burst Fracture

ICD-9: 805.2; 805.2x With spinal cord injury

- **Essentials of Diagnosis**
  - Axial and flexion load to spine with resultant retropulsion of bone into spinal canal; disrupts anterior *and* middle columns (vs anterior column alone in compression fracture); may have a lateral bend, flexion, rotation, or laminar fracture
  - Radiographs show increased interpedicular distance (AP view), kyphotic angulation with or without retropulsion of bone fragments (lateral view); CT scan may help quantify canal compromise and posterior element injury
  - Stable fracture: neurologically intact; posterior column intact (pedicle widening implies posterior arch disruption with instability); <50% anterior body height collapse
  - Unstable fracture: neurologic deficit; loss of 50% vertebral body height; fracture-dislocation; angulation of thoracolumbar junction >20 degrees; canal compromise >30%
  - Disruption of posterior ligamentous complex in anterior column fracture suggests unstable fracture
  - Because injury involves axial compression (eg, fall from a height), incidence of concurrent calcaneal fractures is high

- **Differential Diagnosis**
  - Traumatic vertebral body compression fracture
  - Osteoporotic compression fracture

- **Treatment**
  - Initial: spine precautions; steroids may be indicated if neurologic compromise is present
  - Nonoperative (for most stable and most lumbar burst fractures): rigid orthosis for 4–6 mo; significant remodeling and resorption of fragments is expected
  - Operative (for unstable fractures, stable fracture with >20–30 degrees of kyphosis, any neurologic compromise): primary repair of dural tears; stabilization with or without fusion

- **Pearl**

Progressive neurologic deficit calls for emergent decompression. Long-term outcome of operative fixation of stable fractures is not different from nonoperative treatment.

References

McDonough PW, et al.: The management of acute thoracolumbar burst fractures with anterior corpectomy and Z-plate fixation. Spine 2004;29:1901. [PMID: 15534413]

Wang ST, et al.: Is fusion necessary for surgically treated burst fractures of the thoracolumbar spine?: a prospective, randomized study. Spine 2006;31:2646. [PMID: 17077731]

Spondylolysis & Spondylolisthesis

ICD-9: 738.4

- ■ Essentials of Diagnosis
  - Five types: *type I*—deficiency of the superior facet of S1; *type II*—isthmic, either a defect in the pars interarticularis or an elongation of the pars; *type III*—the degenerative form seen most commonly at L4–L5; *type IV*—traumatic, other than at the pars; *type V*—associated with pathology (eg, neoplasm)
  - Amount of slip is graded by percentages into 4 grades: 0–25%, 26–50%, 51–75%, and 76–100% slip
  - Patients may be asymptomatic or have back or leg pain; young patients may have tight hamstrings and flexed hip and knee gait
  - Radiographs show slip on lateral views and "collar" on "Scotty dog" on oblique views with pars defects present

- ■ Differential Diagnosis
  - Facet syndrome
  - Low back pain (muscular)
  - Spinal stenosis
  - Lumbar disk herniation

- ■ Treatment
  - Grades I and II: treat conservatively with bracing, physical therapy, and activity modification
  - Grades III and IV: at risk for progression; surgical fusion is recommended; most clinicians recommend fusion in situ without correction of the slip because corrective procedures have a higher incidence of neurologic sequelae
  - Epidural steroids can be helpful in treating radicular symptoms
  - Pars repair is an option for patients with normal disks.

- ■ Pearl

Degenerative spondylolisthesis most commonly occurs at the L4–L5 level. There is greater stability at L5–S1, due to the transverse alar ligaments, and L5–S1 is below the level of the iliac crest.

References

Hammerberg KW: New concepts on the pathogenesis and classification of spondylolisthesis. Spine 2005;30(suppl):s4. [PMID: 15767885]

Jacobs WC, et al.: Fusion for low-grade adult isthmic spondylolisthesis: a systematic review of the literature. Eur Spine J 2006;15:391. [PMID: 16217665]

Vibert BT, et al.: Treatment of instability and spondylolisthesis: surgical versus nonsurgical treatment. Clin Orthop 2006;443:222. [PMID: 16462445]

Lumbar Disk Herniation

ICD-9: 722.1.0; 722.73 With radiculopathy or myelopathy

- **■ Essentials of Diagnosis**
  - Often preceded by days or weeks of back pain, indicating damage to annulus around disk; rupture causes pain down leg into nerve root distribution (sciatica in 40% of patients); 90% are L5–S1 or L4–L5 disks
  - L5: weak extensor hallucis longus; decreased sensation in the first web space; posterior tibialis reflex is decreased
  - S1: weak gastrocnemius; decreased sensation in lateral foot; Achilles tendon reflex is decreased
  - L4: weak quadriceps and tibialis anterior; decreased sensation in medial foot, patellar tendon reflex is decreased
  - Positive straight leg raising test for pain down leg; resolves with chronicity or older patients
  - Pain radiating below knee is usually radicular, different from referred pain that stops at knee
  - Radiographs are mandatory, but MRI is exam of choice for diagnosis (positive in 30% of patients without symptoms)

- **■ Differential Diagnosis**
  - Trochanteric bursitis
  - Facet syndrome
  - Tumor in spine
  - Cauda equine syndrome

- **■ Treatment**
  - In >90% of patients, pain resolves by 6 mo with nonsurgical management; in about 50%, symptoms resolve in 1 mo
  - Limited bed rest (1–2 days), analgesics, NSAIDs, and physical therapy; epidural steroid injections may be helpful
  - Surgery has high rate of success in small percentage of patients who fail to respond to conservative care; diskectomy is indicated in patients with unresolved radicular symptoms, tension signs, and radiographic evidence of herniated disk in the same distribution as noted on physical exam

- **■ Pearl**

Patients, especially children, typically have more leg pain than back pain.

References

Awad JN, Moskovich R: Lumbar disc herniations: surgical versus nonsurgical treatment. Clin Orthop 2006;443:183. [PMID: 16462442]

Frino J, et al.: Trends in adolescent lumbar disk herniation. J Pediatr Orthop 2006;26:579. [PMID: 16932094]

Facet Syndrome

ICD-9: 721.3

- **Essentials of Diagnosis**
  - No historical or exam maneuver is unique or specific to facet-mediated low back pain (LBP); in-depth evaluation of neurologic and musculoskeletal systems helps exclude other diagnoses and identify facet joint pathology
  - Pain is worse during extension; can radiate to posterior thigh
  - Plain radiographs, traditionally ordered as the initial step in workup of LBP, determine underlying structural pathologic conditions but are not generally recommended in the first month of symptoms in the absence of significant injury (ie, specific sports injury and fracture)
  - Bone scans are not usually indicated in the initial workup

- **Differential Diagnosis**
  - Lumbosacral disk injuries, diskogenic pain syndrome; or radiculopathy
  - Acute bony injuries of the lumbosacral spine
  - Lumbosacral sprain or strain
  - Lumbosacral spondylolysis or spondylolisthesis
  - Piriformis syndrome
  - Sacroiliac joint injury

- **Treatment**
  - Initial: education, rest, pain relief, maintenance of positions that provide comfort, exercises, and some physical therapy (PT) modalities (ie, ionophoresis, electrical stim); activity modification, rather than bed rest, is strongly recommended because of detrimental effects on bone, connective tissue, muscle, and cardiac function of bed rest beyond 2 days
  - PT: instruction on proper posture and body mechanics in activities of daily living
  - Traction may be helpful
  - Spinal manipulation for both short- and long-term pain relief

- **Pearl**

Patients with LBP who demonstrate red flags (eg, unexplained weight loss, fever, chills) should be evaluated further to rule out malignancy or infection.

References

Slipman CW, et al.: A critical review of the evidence for the use of zygapophysial injections and radiofrequency denervation in the treatment of low back pain. Spine J 2003;3:310. [PMID: 14589192]

Yuan PS, et al.: Nonsurgical and surgical management of lumbar spinal stenosis. Instr Course Lect 2005;54:303. [PMID: 15948458]

Lumbar Spine Stenosis

ICD-9: 724.02

- ■ Essentials of Diagnosis
  - Constriction of the cauda equina roots caused by hypertrophy of the osseous and adjacent soft tissue structures
  - Changes that cause constriction include thickened posterior vertebral elements, presence of osteophytes, thickened ligamentum flavum, or presence of disk herniation
  - Commonly affects middle-aged and elderly patients
  - Patients exhibit claudication that can only be alleviated by flexing the lumbar spine
  - Associated with nonspecific pain in the lower back and lower extremities, difficulty walking, leg paresthesias, and weakness; in severe cases, bladder and bowel incontinence may occur
  - CT and MRI imaging may show narrowing of the lumbar spinal canal with compression of the cauda equina nerve roots

- ■ Differential Diagnosis
  - Vascular claudication
  - Peripheral vascular disease
  - Degenerative spondylolisthesis
  - Epidural abscess
  - Neural compression from metastatic disease to bone
  - Trauma or fracture residua

- ■ Treatment
  - Surgical lumbar decompression is the treatment of choice
  - Evaluate for stability of the spine before and after decompression; if the spine is unstable, fusion is indicated along with decompression
  - Emergent surgical treatment is indicated in patients with bladder or bowel incontinence
  - Conservative medical management with bed rest and pain medication should be reserved for debilitated patients and high-risk surgical patients

- ■ Pearl

Typically, symptoms worsen with ambulation and lessen with sitting or in positions that decrease lumbar lordosis, opening the spinal canal.

References

Aalto TJ, et al.: Pre-operative predictors for postoperative clinical outcome in lumbar stenosis: systematic review. Spine 2006;31:E648. [PMID: 16915081]

Amundsen T, et al.: Lumbar spinal stenosis: conservative or surgical management? A prospective 10-year study. Spine 2000;25:1424. [PMID: 10828926]

Myelodysplasia

ICD-9: 742.9

- ■ Essentials of Diagnosis
  - Neural tube defects result from failure of closure *in utero* and are associated with folic acid deficiency during pregnancy
  - Defects can occur at any level of the spinal cord
  - Progression of severity: *spina bifida*—failure of bony arches to close (skin intact); *meningocele*—meninges exposed; *myelomeningocele*—spinal cord or roots exposed
  - Variable sensory and motor loss, depending on level; areflexia if below L1 (hyperreflexia if above L1) and loss of bowel and bladder control
  - Lesion is static—neurologic function should not deteriorate with increasing age; deterioration suggests tethered cord syndrome, which usually occurs during the growth spurt
  - Hydrocephalus requires a ventriculoperitoneal shunt
  - Foot, knee, and hip deformities are common due to muscle paralysis and imbalance
  - Neuromuscular scoliosis or kyphosis (due to lack of posterior elements) may be present
  - Compare neurologic level on physical exam with historical physical exam findings and roentgenographic studies

- ■ Differential Diagnosis
  - Spinal cord injury

- ■ Treatment
  - Goal: to produce a stable posture for sitting or walking and avoid contractures that would prevent shoe wear, wheel chair use, standing, or walking, depending on the level of neurologic function; function should be maximized
  - Stable posture may require surgical treatment for scoliosis, equinovarus foot deformities, hip dislocation, and hip and knee flexion contractures
  - Ensure adequate urologic follow-up
  - Encourage weight control to improve walking endurance and ability to transfer in patients unable to walk

- ■ Pearl

Latex allergy is potentially catastrophic in these patients. Exposure to latex should be avoided.

References

Guille JT, et al.: Congenital and developmental deformities of the spine in children with myelomeningocele. J Am Acad Orthop Surg 2006;14:294. [PMID: 16675623]

Pilcher J, Sogard L: Myelomeningocele, avocados, and rubber tree plants. Neonatal Netw 2005;24:23. [PMID: 16279052]

Diskitis in Adults

ICD-9: 324.1

- ■ Essentials of Diagnosis
  - May arise from hematogenous spread or from iatrogenic seeding from previous spinal surgery, often in older patients, or immuno-compromised patients
  - Hematogenous spread may occur from any other source of bacteria or fungus in the body (ie, post–colon biopsy; ENT infections; post–dental procedures; endocarditis); patients often are immuno-compromised or IV drug abusers
  - Patients with iatrogenic causes usually present with pain about 1 mo after spinal surgery (presumed direct inoculation); transrectal needle biopsy of the prostate also has been reported to cause diskitis
  - Patients report severe back pain; tension signs may be present
  - Pain with percussion, or paraspinal muscle spasm
  - ESR and CRP may be elevated
  - Radiographs may show endplate erosion and narrowing; bone scan is positive; MRI with gadolinium is usually diagnostic
  - CT-guided biopsy and cultures can help confirm the diagnosis

- ■ Differential Diagnosis
  - Osteomyelitis in the pelvis or lower extremity
  - Recurrent disk
  - Lumbar instability

- ■ Treatment
  - If diskitis is suspected, blood cultures may be helpful; place the patient on bed rest with or without a brace for comfort; perform disk aspiration if constitutional symptoms are present
  - If no culture is obtained, give empiric IV antibiotics for 6 wk
  - If the diskitis is unresponsive to IV antibiotics or an abscess develops, surgical debridement and irrigation is indicated

- ■ Pearl

The diagnosis of disk space infection is easy to miss because patients with back pain may have a lot of pain after surgery. Similarly, many older, immunocompromised patients with infection located elsewhere will have back pain.

References

Saeed MU, et al.: Anaerobic spondylodiscitis: case series and systematic review. South Med J 2005;98:144. [PMID: 15759942]

Tasdemiroglu E, et al.: Iatrogenic spondylodiscitis. Case report and review of the literature. Neurosurg Focus 2004;16:ECP1. [PMID: 15202880]

4

Neoplasms

ICD-9 Codes for Bone, Connective, & Soft Tissue Tumors

Malignant Neoplasms of Bone and Articular Cartilage: 170

Bones of the skull and face	170.0
Mandible	170.1
Vertebral column	170.2
Ribs, sternum, and clavicle	170.3
Scapula and long bones of upper limb	170.4
Short bones of upper limb	170.5
Pelvic bones, sacrum, and coccyx	170.6
Long bones of lower limb	170.7
Short bones of lower limb	170.8
Sites unspecified	170.9

Malignant Neoplasms of Connective Tissue and Other Soft Tissues: 171 (includes muscle, tendon, synovium, and fat)

Head, face, and neck	171.0
Upper limb (including shoulder)	171.2
Lower limb (including hip)	171.3
Thorax	171.4
Abdomen	171.5
Pelvis	171.6
Trunk	171.7
Overlapping sites of origins	171.8
Sites unspecified	171.9

Benign Neoplasms of Bone and Articular Cartilage: 213

Bones of skull and face	213.0
Mandible	213.1
Vertebral column	213.2
Ribs, sternum, and clavicle	213.3
Scapula and long bones of upper limb	213.4
Short bones of upper limb	213.5
Pelvic bones, sacrum, and coccyx	213.6
Long bones of lower limb	213.7
Short bones of lower limb	213.8
Sites unspecified	213.9

Lipoma: 214

Skin and subcutaneous face	214.0
Other skin and subcutaneous tissue	214.1
Overlapping sites	214.8
Site unspecified	214.9

Benign Neoplasms of Connective and Other Soft Tissues: 215

Head, face, and neck	215.0
Upper limb (including shoulder)	215.2
Lower limb (including hip)	215.3
Thorax	215.4
Abdomen	215.5
Pelvis	215.6
Trunk	215.7
Overlapping sites of origins	215.8
Sites unspecified	215.9

Evaluation & Staging of Tumors

ICD-9: not applicable

■ Essentials of Diagnosis

- Aims of surgical staging: to determine the surgical margins of resection and to facilitate interinstitutional and interdisciplinary communication regarding treatment data and results
- Enneking system of surgical staging of bone and soft tissue tumors is based on grade (G), site (T), and metastasis (M) and uses histologic, radiologic, and clinical criteria; it is the most widely used staging system and has been adopted by the Musculoskeletal Tumor Society
- *Grade:* G0—benign lesion; G1—low-grade malignant lesion; G2—high-grade malignant lesion
- Site: T0—benign intracapsular and intracompartmental lesion; T1—intracompartmental lesion; T2—extracompartmental lesion
- Metastasis: M0—no regional or distant metastasis; M1—regional or distant metastasis
- CT has a role in the evaluation of local disease in detail and in assessing the lungs for pulmonary metastases
- MRI allows accurate depiction of the soft tissues for sensitive detection of soft tissue tumor extension and medullary involvement
- Radionuclide bone scanning has a role in detecting metastases, skip lesions, lesion multiplicity, and postoperative tumor recurrence

■ Differential Diagnosis

- Benign lesion to high-grade malignant lesion
- Intracapsular lesion to extracompartmental lesion
- Metastasis or no metastasis

■ Treatment

- Aims of limb salvage surgery: to cure the disease and to preserve limb function for the patient; achieved by using a combination of limb salvage surgery and adjuvant therapy

■ Pearl

Radiography is the initial imaging modality in the evaluation of bone tumors. Some benign lesions have characteristic radiographic features that make biopsy unnecessary.

References

Pommersheim WJ, Chew FS: Imaging, diagnosis, and staging of bone tumors: a primer. Semin Roentgenol 2004;39:361. [PMID: 15372750]

Stacy GS, et al.: Staging of bone tumors: a review with illustrative examples. AJR Am J Roentgenol 2006;186:967. [PMID: 16554565]

Benign Tumors in Bone

ICD-9: 213.x

- Essentials of Diagnosis
  - Benign bone tumors often are asymptomatic
  - Soft tissue tumors usually present as a mass without pain
  - All suspected musculoskeletal neoplasms require radiographs
  - Appearance and location of mass on radiographs are keys to diagnosis
  - Historical course of the tumor is significant: slow growth is indicative of a benign process
  - *Stage 1*: "latent"; usually asymptomatic; may resolve without treatment; observation is appropriate
  - *Stage 2*: "active"; not likely to resolve; surgical intervention is usually indicated
  - *Stage 3*: "aggressive"; not malignant but recurrence is likely and aggressive treatment is indicated

- Differential Diagnosis
  - Nonossifying fibroma
  - Unicameral cyst
  - Osteoblastoma
  - Aneurysmal bone cyst
  - Osteoid osteoma
  - Osteochondroma
  - Giant cell tumor (occasionally aggressive)

- Treatment
  - Depends on the staging of the individual lesion
  - Surgery may be indicated to prevent fracture or resect the tumor

- Pearl

If a biopsy is warranted, it should be performed by the orthopaedic surgeon who would perform the resection.

References

Geniets C, et al.: Proceedings of the European Society of Musculoskeletal Radiology (ESSR) training module, Antwerp, 20-21.01.05. Part two: bone tumors. Benign bone lesions: characteristic imaging features. JBR-BTR 2006;89:266. [PMID: 17147017]

Pommersheim WJ, Chew FS: Imaging, diagnosis and staging of bone tumors: a primer. Semin Roentgenol 2004;39:361. [PMID: 15372750]

Bone Infarct

ICD-9: 733.4

- ■ Essentials of Diagnosis
  - Area of ischemic death in the metaphysis or epiphysis
  - Causes: idiopathic; secondary to increased alcohol consumption, corticosteroid use, trauma, or renal transplantation; associated with increased endogenous steroid levels, as in patients with Cushing syndrome, and with hemoglobinopathies (eg, sickle cell disease)
  - Metaphyseal is most common; occurs around the knee, hip, and shoulder; produces a sclerotic honeycombed pattern
  - Epiphyseal occurs at the femoral condyles and proximal femoral and humeral epiphyses; produces a lytic lesion
  - CT, MRI, or bone scan is useful in confirming the diagnosis

- ■ Differential Diagnosis
  - Tumor: metaphyseal (low-grade cartilaginous tumor, enchondroma); epiphyseal (chondroblastoma)
  - Calcium pyrophosphate deposition disease
  - Osteochondritis dissecans
  - Stress fracture

- ■ Treatment
  - Rule out treatable etiology
  - Evaluate benefits of conservative management versus surgical intervention (decompression, bone graft, total joint arthroplasty, joint fusion) in symptomatic cases

- ■ Pearl

Bone infarcts may mimic bone tumors and frequently are found around the knee as an incidental finding.

Reference

Gould CF et al.: Bone Tumor mimics: avoiding misdiagnosis. Curr Prob Diagn Radiol. 2007;36:124. [PMID: 17484955]

Benign Chondroid-Forming Tumors

ICD-9: 213.x

- **Essentials of Diagnosis**
  - Cartilage tumors have a characteristic radiographic appearance, demonstrating flecks of calcified cartilage; they are slow-growing with a geographic lysis and central calcification
  - *Chondroblastoma*: a lesion of the epiphysis of childhood; malignant transformation is rare
  - *Enchondroma*: common, centrally located chondroma of bone; 50% occur in the hands or feet
  - *Osteochondroma*: second most common benign tumor of bone; arises from a defect in the outer edge of the growth plate on the metaphyseal side and results in a bony exostosis with a cartilage cap that always points away from the joint of origin; usually palpable near joints
  - Often found on radiographs as an incidental finding after minor trauma; enchondroma may present as a pathologic fracture

- **Differential Diagnosis**
  - Chondrosarcoma
  - Osteosarcoma with chondroblastic features
  - Bone infarct
  - Chondromyxoid fibroma
  - Multiple osteochondromatosis
  - Multiple enchondromatosis (Ollier disease)

- **Treatment**
  - Most chondroid-forming tumors are benign lesions and can be managed conservatively
  - Symptomatic osteochondroma lesions can be excised to alleviate pain, improve joint motion, prevent deformity, and relieve impingement on tendons, nerves, or vessels
  - Enchondromas can be treated with curettage and bone grafting to restore strength to bone after healing from a pathologic fracture

- **Pearl**

The most common bony lesion found in the hand is the enchondroma.

Reference

O'Connor MI, Bancroft LW: Benign and malignant cartilage tumors of the hand. Hand Clin 2004;20:317. [PMID: 15275690]

Benign Fibrous Tumors of the Bone

ICD-9: 733.29 Fibrous dysplasia; 213.x

- ### Essentials of Diagnosis

  - Affect metaphysis of long bones; most common are fibrous cortical defect, nonossifying fibroma, and fibrous dysplasia (FD); often incidental findings on radiographs
  - Characteristic radiographic appearance—slow growing, lytic interior, sclerotic margin; larger tumors may be multiloculated; radiographs are diagnostic, obviating need for biopsy
  - *Fibrous cortical defect* (ages 2–20 y): produces spindle-shaped cells in storiform pattern; radiograph (usually an incidental finding) shows well-demarcated lesion, sclerotic border, usually 1–2 cm
  - *Nonossifying fibroma*: basically a larger fibrous cortical defect; loculated radiographic appearance with sclerotic borders, may expand cortex due to slow growth; if risk of fracture (>50% of cortex, or painful, in a child >10 y), perform surgery with curettage and bone graft
  - *FD* (typically diagnosed in first 3 decades): normal bone and marrow is replaced by fibrous tissue from which small, woven spicules of bone arise; caused by mutations in osteoblast cell line; patient may be sexually precocious (McCune-Albright syndrome), have abnormal skin pigmentation or thyroid disease; radiograph shows lucent area appearing fine and granular-like ground glass; cortex may expand and thin, and deformity or fracture may occur; may be polyostotic

- ### Differential Diagnosis

  - Cortical desmoid
  - Solitary bone cyst
  - Chondromyxoid fibroma

- ### Treatment

  - Except for FD, treatment is expectant unless fracture prophylaxis is necessary; tumors are treated with curettage and bone graft when necessary; for patients with FD, bisphosphonates can reduce symptoms, but intramedullary fixation and cortical strut grafting may be needed to prevent or correct deformities

- ### Pearl

FD commonly occurs in the proximal femur or hip, fibrous cortical defect in the distal femoral metaphysis.

References

DiCaprio MR, Enneking WF: Fibrous dysplasia. J Bone Joint Surg Am 2005;87:1848. [PMID: 16085630]

Jackson WF, et al.: Early management of pathological fractures in children. Injury 2007;38:194. [PMID: 17054958]

Benign Osteoid-Forming Tumors

ICD-9: 213.x

- **Essentials of Diagnosis**
  - Most common types are osteoid osteoma, osteoblastoma, osteochondroma, and multiple osteochondromatosis
  - Characteristic radiographic appearance: usually a well-defined geographic lesion, with a sclerotic reactive margin; some lytic component may be seen, but histology shows osteoblastic activity; cortex may be expanded, indicating slow growth
  - *Osteoid osteoma* (young males aged 0–30 y): cortical sclerosis on radiographs and possibly a lytic nidus a few mm in size; pain is worse at night and relieved by NSAIDs; deformities may occur; bone scan and CT are useful in diagnosis
  - *Osteoblastoma*: a large osteoid osteoma with a propensity for posterior elements of the spine; more common in males
  - *Osteochondroma*: cartilaginous tumor that develops during rapid skeletal growth (see Benign Chondroid-Forming Tumors); usually biopsy is required for diagnosis of sarcomatous change but diagnosis is clear from radiographs in most cases
  - *Multiple osteochondromatosis*: osteochondromas of many bones; familial form (hereditary multiple exostoses) is autosomal dominant

- **Differential Diagnosis**
  - Osteosarcoma
  - Chondrosarcoma

- **Treatment**
  - *Osteoid osteoma*: NSAIDs for diagnosis and symptom relief; excision of nidus for permanent relief—may need CT localization; radiofrequency ablation with CT guidance is an option
  - *Osteoblastoma*: can be treated with curettage and possible bone graft for cord or nerve root compromise, or for concern for fracture or pain relief; radiation therapy may be helpful in certain cases near the cord

- **Pearl**

Because osteoid osteoma is a vascular tumor, substances that cause vasodilation (eg, alcohol) may precipitate an acute pain episode.

References

Ozaki T, et al.: Osteoid osteoma and osteoblastoma of the spine: experiences with 22 patients. Clin Orthop Relat Res 2002;394. [PMID: 11953633]

Zileli M, et al.: Osteoid osteomas and osteoblastomas of the spine. Neurosurg Focus 2003;15:E5. [PMID: 15323462]

Benign Cyst-Forming Tumors

ICD-9: 213.x

- **Essentials of Diagnosis**

  - Most common types are simple (unicameral) bone cyst (SBC), aneurysmal bone cyst (ABC), and epidermoid cyst
  - Characteristic radiographic appearance: usually lytic and metaphyseal, with a pseudoloculated appearance, and marked thinning of the adjacent cortical bone; the cortex, while thinned, may be expanded, indicating slow growth
  - *SBC*: occurs in children aged 5–15 y; may first be seen after pathologic fracture; fracture heals normally and may heal lesion
  - *ABC*: hemorrhagic lesion with characteristics of a giant cell tumor; most patients are 10–20-y old and female; femur is most commonly affected
  - *Epidermoid cyst*: occurs in the phalanges due to traumatic implantation of nail bed epithelium into the bone

- **Differential Diagnosis**

  - Giant cell tumor (ABC)
  - Chondromyxoid fibroma (ABC)
  - Fibrous dysplasia (SBC)
  - Hemorrhagic osteosarcoma (ABC)
  - Enchondroma (epidermoid cyst)

- **Treatment**

  - *SBCs*: aggressive treatment in lower extremity or to prevent pathologic fracture; steroid or bone marrow injection into lesion after aspiration 3–5 times at intervals of 2–3 mo is often effective; curettage and bone grafting is an option
  - *ABCs*: can be treated by curettage and bone grafting; low-dose radiotherapy may be indicated for incompletely resected, recurrent, or aggressive cysts

- **Pearl**

Solitary bone cyst is the most common cause of pathologic fracture in children.

References

Kanellopoulos AD, et al.: Percutaneous reaming of simple bone cysts in children followed by injection of demineralized bone matrix and autologous bone marrow. J Pediatr Orthop 2005;25:671. [PMID: 16199953]

Mendenhall WM, et al.: Aneurysmal bone cyst. Am J Clin Oncol 2006;29:311. [PMID: 12063325]

Rougraff BT, Kling TJ: Treatment of active unicameral bone cysts with percutaneous injection of demineralized bone matrix and autogenous bone marrow. J Bone Joint Surg Am 2002;84A:921. [PMID: 16755186]

Giant Cell Tumor of Bone

ICD-9: 213.x

- ■ Essentials of Diagnosis
  - Although many bone tumors contain giant cells, the benign giant cell tumor of bone affects adults (females more than males) and constitutes ~5–10% of all benign bone tumors
  - ~50% of lesions occur around the knee
  - Associated with overexpression of osteoprotegerin ligand, which stimulates osteoclast differentiation
  - Lytic lesion, in the metaphyseal area that may grow into the joint surface area
  - Small chance of metastasis to the lung
  - Pain is the usual presenting symptom but the tumor may present as an incidental finding or a pathologic fracture

- ■ Differential Diagnosis
  - Aneurysmal bone cyst
  - Osteosarcoma
  - Chondroblastoma
  - Infection (mycobacterial or fungal)

- ■ Treatment
  - Because of the chance of metastasis, pulmonary staging is important, as well as aggressive curettage, followed by a secondary treatment to minimize the chance of recurrence
  - Adjuvant treatment possibilities include high-speed burring, with phenol, peroxide, or liquid nitrogen; the lesion is then packed with bone cement
  - Recurrence mandates even more aggressive en bloc resection and reconstruction
  - Surgically unresectable lesions can be treated with moderate-dose radiation (45–50 Gy)

- ■ Pearl

Bone lysis around the bone cement is suggestive of recurrence.

References

Mendenhall WM, et al.: Giant cell tumor of bone. Am J Clin Oncol 2006;29:96. [PMID: 16462511]

Turcotte RE: Giant cell tumor of bone. Orthop Clin North Am 2006;37:35. [PMID: 16311110]

Chondroid-Forming Sarcomas

ICD-9: 170.x Malignant; 213.x Benign

- **Essentials of Diagnosis**
  - Chondrosarcoma comprises a heterogenous group of cartilage-based neoplasms—including primary, secondary, dedifferentiated, clear cell, and mesenchymal—that are less common and less aggressive than osteosarcoma
  - Most often occur in patients aged 30–60 y
  - Tumors are commonly low grade and grow to large sizes but rarely metastasize
  - Pain is minimal but is frequently the presenting symptom
  - Secondary chondrosarcoma generally arises in patients with multiple hereditary exostoses

- **Differential Diagnosis**
  - Osteosarcoma with chondroblastic features
  - Enchondroma
  - Bone infarct

- **Treatment**
  - Because these are generally low-grade tumors, they do not respond well to radiation or chemotherapy
  - Surgical excision is the best treatment option
  - Low-grade chondrosarcomas are unlikely to recur after wide excision
  - High-grade chondrosarcomas have a higher recurrence rate and can metastasize to the lungs; amputation should be considered
  - Five-year survival rate in patients treated for chondrosarcoma is 50–75%

- **Pearl**

The cornerstone to diagnosis of chondrosarcoma is the absence of osteoid formation.

References

Terek RM: Recent advances in the basic science of chondrosarcoma. Orthop Clin North Am 2006;37:9. [PMID: 16311107]

Weiner SD: Enchondroma and chondrosarcoma of bone: clinical, radiologic, and histologic differentiation. Instr Course Lect 2004;53:645. [PMID: 15116654]

Osteosarcoma

ICD-9: 170.x

- **Essentials of Diagnosis**
  - Primary tumor of bone characterized by formation of osteoid, occurring in the second or third decade, more commonly in males
  - Various forms: classic; parosteal (on the metaphyseal surface of the bone with no medullary component); periosteal (also on the surface but tends to be more diaphyseal); telangiectatic or hemorrhagic; secondary (arising from osteoblastoma, Paget disease, giant cell tumor, fibrous dysplasia); intramedullary; radiation induced; multicentric; and soft-tissue
  - ~50% of lesions occur around the knee
  - Short history of swelling and pain, often worse at night
  - Radiographs show mixed lytic and blastic lesion, aggressive with indistinct margins, "sunburst" appearance

- **Differential Diagnosis**
  - Infection
  - Benign giant cell tumor
  - Aneurysmal bone cyst
  - Chondroma

- **Treatment**
  - Careful staging and biopsy results form the basis for treatment plan
  - Based on the histologic picture, preoperative adjuvant chemotherapy may shrink the tumor and allow limb-salvage surgery
  - High (>90%) tumor necrosis at definitive limb salvage surgery portends a good 5-year survival rate
  - Amputation is reserved for the exceptional or recurrent case

- **Pearl**

Parosteal and periosteal forms are usually low-grade tumors with a good long-term survival rate.

References

Klein MJ, Siegal GP: Osteosarcoma: anatomic and histologic variants. Am J Clin Pathol 2006;125:555. [PMID: 16627266]

Marina N, et al.: Biology and therapeutic advances for pediatric osteosarcoma. Oncologist 2004;9:422. [PMID: 15266096]

Myeloma

ICD-9: 203 Multiple; 238.6 Monostotic

- Essentials of Diagnosis
  - Most common primary tumor of bone characterized by malignant monoclonal plasma cells, punched-out boney lesions, and a monoclonal gammopathy
  - May present as pathologic fracture
  - 90% of cases occur after age 40 y
  - Most lesions are in the axial skeleton and the proximal humerus and femur
  - History of pain with fatigue and weakness
  - Radiographic appearance: punched-out, lytic lesions with typically no blastic sclerotic response; indistinct margins; may just cause diffuse osteopenia

- Differential Diagnosis
  - Solitary plasmacytoma
  - Lymphoma
  - Metastatic disease
  - Aneurysmal bone cyst
  - Hyperparathyroidism

- Treatment
  - Primary treatment is chemotherapy
  - Skeletal complications may be reduced by using bisphosphonates
  - Local treatment is the same as for metastatic disease, with cemented intramedullary devices and prosthetic components, followed by irradiation; bleeding can be extensive

- Pearl

Lesions distal to the knee and elbow are rare, and a bone survey is necessary to see other lesions; a bone scan is not helpful.

References

Lacy MQ, et al.: Mayo clinic consensus statement for the use of bisphosphonates in multiple myeloma. Mayo Clin Proc 2006;81:1047. [PMID: 16901028]

Yeh HS, Berenson JR: Myeloma bone disease and treatment options. Eur J Cancer 2006;42:1554. [PMID 16797971]

Hemangioma

ICD-9: 228.0

- **Essentials of Diagnosis**
  - Benign vascular tumor of superficial cutaneous or deep intramuscular tissue or bone
  - *Several types*: *solitary capillary hemangioma* occurs after birth and usually regresses over years; *cavernous hemangioma* is larger, with vascular spaces that give it a grapelike appearance; *arteriovenous hemangioma* causes shunting with a bruit, thrill, and increased temperature
  - Cavernous hemangioma is asymptomatic until intralesional hemorrhage occurs, either spontaneously or after minor trauma

- **Differential Diagnosis**
  - Klippel-Trenaunay-Weber syndrome
  - Malignant melanoma
  - Kaposi sarcoma
  - Maffucci syndrome
  - Metastatic carcinoma

- **Treatment**
  - Steroid treatment, intralesionally and topically
  - Vascular embolization may be beneficial but observation for compartment syndrome is necessary
  - Surgical removal is necessary if significant arteriovenous shunting occurs

- **Pearl**

Hemangiomas of infancy require special attention to ensure that no associated deformities are present.

References

Akgun I, et al.: Intra-articular hemangioma of the knee. Arthroscopy 2003;19:E17. [PMID: 12627134]

Waldt S, et al.: Imaging of benign and malignant soft tissue masses of the foot. Eur Radiol 2003;13:1125. [PMID: 12695837]

Synovial Cell Sarcoma

ICD-9: 171.x; (Morphology: M9040/3)

- ■ Essentials of Diagnosis
  - Fourth most common soft tissue sarcoma
  - Age range is 15–35 y
  - Male-to-female ratio is slightly >1
  - Initially slow growing; may be associated with an injury and have dystrophic calcification
  - Only 10% occur in a major joint; tumors arise in juxta-articular areas, especially around the knee
  - Pain is present in 50% of patients
  - Radiographic findings may include calcified opacities or hetero-topic bone

- ■ Differential Diagnosis
  - Extraskeletal chondrosarcoma
  - Rhabdomyosarcoma
  - Fibrosarcoma

- ■ Treatment
  - Complete wide excision with chemotherapy, to which the tumor is frequently quite sensitive
  - Prognosis is related to size of lesion, male sex, truncal location of the tumor, age of the patient (age >20 y at time of diagnosis implies worse prognosis), and response to first-line chemotherapy

- ■ Pearl

A lower risk of adverse outcome is associated with a tumor size <5 cm, age <20–25 y, and a well-differentiated histologic picture.

Reference

Spurrell EL, et al.: Prognostic factors in advanced synovial sarcoma: an analysis of 104 patients treated at the Royal Marsden Hospital. Ann Oncol 2005;16:437. [PMID: 15653701]

Marjolin Ulcer (Squamous Cell Carcinoma Arising from Chronic Osteomyelitis)

ICD-9: 170.x; 238; (Morphology: M8070/3)

- **Essentials of Diagnosis**
  - Metaplasia of the sinus tract in chronic osteomyelitis can lead to squamous cell carcinoma (SCC)
  - Long-term draining sinus tract must be present for SCC to develop; chronic purulent drainage causes continuous degeneration and metaplasia of the epithelialized lining of the sinus tract
  - 0.23–1.3% of all chronic osteomyelitis results in SCC
  - Symptoms may include worsening pain, enlarging mass, or a change in the character or consistency of the draining fluid; however, characteristic findings may be absent
  - Radiologic images may show a lytic lesion in the affected area; however, images can appear unchanged
  - Histologic appearance is of a well-differentiated keratinizing squamous cell carcinoma
  - Diagnosis is confirmed by biopsy, which is indicated for any wound that has been open for ≥10 y

- **Differential Diagnosis**
  - Chronic osteomyelitis
  - Cutaneous ulcers
  - Chronic sinus tract

- **Treatment**
  - Surgical treatment includes removal of the tumor and en bloc resection of the affected bone
  - The sinus tract must be removed with clear margins

- **Pearl**

A sinus tract or long-term, nonhealing wound must be present, usually for years, before SCC develops.

References

Eltorai IM, et al.: Marjolin's ulcer in patients with spinal cord injury. J Spinal Cord Med 2002;25:191. [PMID: 12214906]

Enoch S, et al.: Early diagnosis is vital in the management of squamous cell carcinomas associated with chronic non healing ulcers: a case series and review of the literature. Int Wound J 2004;1:165. [PMID: 16722875]

Ewing Sarcoma

ICD-9: 171.x; (Morphology: M9260/3)

- Essentials of Diagnosis
  - Rare disease in which malignant cells are found in the bone of children and young adults (ages 5–25 y, most often teenagers); categorized as a *primitive neuroectodermal tumor* (PNET)
  - Most common areas are the pelvis, femur, humerus, and ribs
  - Pain occurs at the site of the tumor and, occasionally, swelling; fever can occur
  - Skeletal radiographs show a metaphyseal-diaphyseal lesion with lysis and permeative destruction with an onion-skin effect on the periosteum
  - Workup includes chest radiograph, CT scan of chest, and bone scan prior to biopsy of the tumor

- Differential Diagnosis
  - Chondrosarcoma
  - Eosinophilic granuloma, skeletal
  - Lymphoma
  - Osteomyelitis (acute or chronic)
  - Osteosarcoma

- Treatment
  - Depends on where the cancer is located, how far it has spread, stage of disease, and age and general health of the patient
  - Alternatives include combination chemotherapy; surgery and combination chemotherapy; radiation therapy and combination chemotherapy

- Pearl

Because of the limited prognosis in patients with metastases, high diagnostic accuracy in morphologic imaging methods, functional procedures, and histologic analyses is essential to permit early identification of the tumor.

Reference

Bernstein M, et al.: Ewing's sarcoma family of tumors: current management. Oncologist 2006;11:503. [PMID: 16720851]

Fibrosarcoma of Bone

ICD-9: 170.x; (Morphology: M8810/3)

- ■ Essentials of Diagnosis
  - Can be diagnosed in patients of any age, but more common in those in the fourth decade of life
  - Usually occurs in the lower extremities, especially the femur and tibia
  - Usually presents as a painful mass
  - Radiologic appearance is that of an osteolytic lesion; radiographs show a poorly defined, destructive, radiolucent lesion of the metaphysis
  - Early radiologic picture shows a distinct, well-defined margin; in advanced disease, there is a poorly marginated and permeative lesion with bony destruction
  - MRI helps define intraosseous spread and soft tissue extension; bone scan demonstrates increased uptake

- ■ Differential Diagnosis
  - Leiomyosarcoma
  - Metastatic carcinoma
  - Melanoma
  - Malignant fibrous histiocytoma
  - Multiple myeloma
  - Infection

- ■ Treatment
  - Treatment includes radical surgical excision and adjuvant radiation therapy
  - Limb salvage excision with wide margins is indicated for early disease
  - Moderate disease require radical or wide margins with adjuvant chemotherapy or radiation therapy
  - Prognosis depends on histologic grade

- ■ Pearl

Fibrosarcoma can present in the diaphysis of long bones—an uncommon location for most bone tumors.

Reference

Papagelopoulos PJ, et al.: Clinicopathological features, diagnosis and treatment of fibrosarcoma of bone. Am J Orthop 2002;31:253. [PMID: 12041516]

Liposarcoma

ICD-9: 170.x; (Morphology: M8850/3)

- ■ Essentials of Diagnosis
  - • Second most common malignant tumor of soft tissue (first is malignant fibrous histiocytoma)
  - • Usually occurs in older adults (>40 y)
  - • Presents as a mass with well-defined boundaries in the retroperitoneum, buttock, or thigh; not usually painful
  - • Five histologic subtypes: well-differentiated, dedifferentiated, myxoid, pleomorphic, and mixed
  - • Most common types are well-differentiated and myxoid; these grow slowly and recur locally
  - • Pleomorphic liposarcomas are fast growing and may be painful; survival is poor due to metastasis
  - • Difficult to differentiate from lipomas; the presence of thick septa and associated nonadipose masses on imaging increases the likelihood that the tumor is a liposarcoma

- ■ Differential Diagnosis
  - • Lipoma
  - • Malignant fibrous histiocytoma

- ■ Treatment
  - • Wide local excision is usual but aggressiveness correlates with histologic grade, so more radical surgical treatment and chemotherapy may be indicated for patients with high-grade lesions

- ■ Pearl

Liposarcoma is more likely (13–32-fold) with male sex and the presence of thick septa and associated nonadipose masses on imaging.

References

Kransdorf MJ, et al.: Imaging of fatty tumors: distinction of lipoma and well-differentiated liposarcoma. Radiology 2002;224:99. [PMID: 12091667]

Mankin HJ, Hornicek FJ: Diagnosis, classification, and management of soft tissue sarcomas. Cancer Control 2005;12:5. [PMID: 15668648]

Murphey MD, et al.: From the archives of the AFIP: imaging of musculoskeletal liposarcoma with radiologic-pathologic correlation. Radiographics 2005;25:1371. [PMID: 16160117]

Chondrosarcoma, Extraskeletal

ICD-9: 170.x; (Morphology: M9220/3)

■ Essentials of Diagnosis

- Rare malignant tumor of cartilage in which the cancer matrix is entirely chondroid in composition
- Gradual age-related increase in incidence, with peak occurring in sixth and seventh decades
- Male-to-female ratio is equal
- Frequently occurs (80% of cases) in deep soft tissue of the lower extremity and buttock
- Pain is the presenting symptom; pain is described as dull, aching, and intermittent; may be severe at night
- Radiographic findings include discrete calcified opacities, a hallmark of cartilage lesions; presents as radiolucency with mostly distributed punctate or ring-like opacities
- Metastases are frequent in patients with high-grade lesions and are more frequent than skeletal chondrosarcoma

■ Differential Diagnosis

- Enchondroma
- Calcifying aponeurotic fibroma
- Myxoid liposarcoma
- Mixed tumor of soft tissue

■ Treatment

- Complete wide excision; surgery is the primary and most successful treatment option
- Others options, including irradiation and chemotherapy, play a minor role and usually apply to high-grade lesions, only
- Prognosis is related to size of lesion, anatomic location, and histologic grade

■ Pearl

The peak incidence of chondrosarcoma is in patients >50 y.

References

Antonescu CR, et al.: Skeletal and extraskeletal myxoid chondrosarcoma: a comparative clinicopathologic, ultrastructural, and molecular study. Cancer 1998;83:1504. [PMID: 9781944]

Hisaoka M, Hashimoto H: Extraskeletal myxoid chondrosarcoma: updated clinicopathological and molecular genetic characteristics. Pathol Int 2005;55:453. [PMID: 15998372]

Malignant Fibrous Histiocytoma

ICD-9: 171.x; (Morphology: M8830/3)

- Essentials of Diagnosis
  - Comprise about 5% of bone tumors
  - More common in fourth and fifth decades and in male patients
  - Predilection for the same sites as fibrosarcoma or osteosarcoma (ie, the knee is a prime site)
  - Secondary tumors can arise from preexisting benign lesions, such as bone infarcts, or previous radiation therapy
  - Geographic lysis, with cortical destruction, is seen on radiographs, with little reactive bone

- Differential Diagnosis
  - Fibrosarcoma
  - Myeloma

- Treatment
  - Treatment mirrors that for high-grade fibrosarcoma: aggressive wide resection and adjuvant chemotherapy
  - Prognosis is poor

- Pearl

This diagnosis became popular in the 1960s and 1970s, but subsequent investigation has shown that the cells are not derived from histiocytic cells, but are more accurately diagnosed as subtypes of other sarcomas.

References

Erlandson RA, Antonescu CR: The rise and fall of malignant fibrous histiocytoma. Ultrastruct Pathol 2004;28:283. [PMID: 15764577]

Randall RL, et al.: Malignant fibrous histiocytoma of soft tissue: an abandoned diagnosis. Am J Orthop 2004;33:602. [PMID: 15641745]

Metastatic Disease Management

ICD-9: 198.5

- ■ Essentials of Diagnosis
  - The spine is the most frequent site of bone metastasis
  - Carcinomas that commonly spread to bone are prostate, breast, kidney, thyroid, and lung
  - Hypercalcemia and normochromic normocytic anemia may be present
  - Pain is a common presenting complaint, if pathologic fracture has not occurred
  - Blastic lesions are less likely to cause pathologic fractures
  - Biopsy *usually* is helpful in diagnosis of the primary tumor

- ■ Differential Diagnosis
  - Infection
  - Aneurysmal bone cyst
  - Hyperparathyroidism
  - Myeloma

- ■ Treatment
  - Goals are to alleviate pain and prevent pathologic fracture
  - Bisphosphonates are part of the multimodal approach to managing metastatic disease
  - Operative treatment is not warranted unless the projected life expectancy is at least 6 wk; local treatment is surgical intervention with cemented intramedullary devices and prosthetic components, followed by irradiation

- ■ Pearl

The differential diagnosis of any bone lesion in a patient >40 y must include metastatic disease and infection.

References

Clines GA, Guise TA: Hypercalcaemia of malignancy and basic research on mechanisms responsible for osteolytic and osteoblastic metastasis to bone. Endocr Relat Cancer 2005;12:549. [PMID: 16172192]

Selvaggi G, Scagliotti GV: Management of bone metastases in cancer: a review. Crit Rev Oncol Hematol 2005;56:365. [PMID: 15978828]

Weber KL, et al.: An approach to the management of the patient with metastatic bone disease. Instr Course Lect 2004;53:663. [PMID: 15116657]

Adult Joint Problems & Reconstruction

Hemiarthroplasty Problem Evaluation

ICD-9: 996.4 (Mechanical complication of internal orthopedic device)

- ■ Essential Concepts
  - • Hemiarthroplasty refers to replacement of one side of a diarthrodial joint; it is commonly used for displaced fractures of the femoral neck, 3- or 4-part proximal humerus fractures that are not amenable to open fracture treatment, and tumor treatment; shoulder hemiarthroplasty is used to treat shoulder arthritis in patients with a rotator cuff tear
  - • Problems and complications, and associated symptoms, include:
  - • *Infection*: acute or chronic onset of pain, suspicious for infection with elevated CRP and ESR; WBC count may be normal; radiographs are not helpful; diagnosis is confirmed by aspiration
  - • *Dislocation*: ~3.4% rate of dislocation, usually within a few weeks of initial surgery; acute onset of pain when dislocation occurs; diagnosis is confirmed by radiographs
  - • *Degeneration of residual joint surface*: gradual onset of pain, accentuated with use of the extremity, minimal rest pain; cartilage thinning on radiographs; diagnosis is confirmed by culture-negative aspiration and positive response to pain relief with lidocaine injection
  - • *Disarticulation of prosthesis*: prosthesis comes apart with acute pain, inability to use the extremity; diagnosis is apparent on radiographs
  - • *Periprosthetic fracture*: usually obvious on radiographic evaluation

- ■ Essentials of Management
  - • Treatment is specific to the problem: for infection, debride or remove prosthesis; for dislocation, perform closed or possibly open reduction; for degeneration, surgically replace remaining joint surface; for disarticulation, perform surgical replacement; for periprosthetic fracture, surgical reduction or replacement with long stem femoral or humeral component

- ■ Pearl

Constant pain and night pain suggest infection.

References

Bhandari M, et al.: Internal fixation compared with arthroplasty for displaced fractures of the femoral neck. A meta-analysis. J Bone Joint Surg Am 2003; 85-A:1673. [PMID: 12954824]

Georgiou G, et al.: Dissociation of bipolar hemiarthroplasty of the hip after dislocation. A report of five different cases and review of literature. Injury 2006;37:162. [PMID: 16420955]

Total Hip Arthroplasty: Painful

ICD-9: V54.8 Hip replacement after care; 719.45 Hip pain

- **Essential Concepts**
  - Total hip arthroplasty is the surgical treatment of end-stage inflammatory or degenerative arthritis of the hip, performed by replacing the articular surfaces of the acetabulum and the femur
  - Prosthesis: various materials are used (ie, metal, polyethylene, ceramic); usually there are 2 femoral components, a head and a stem, and at least 2 acetabular components, a metal shell and a plastic or ceramic liner; polymethylmethacrylate cement may be used to fix the prosthesis to bone
  - Problems, and associated symptoms, include:
  - *Infection*: acute onset or chronic pain, suspicious for infection with elevated CRP and ESR; WBC count may be normal and patient afebrile; wound may or may not be inflamed; diagnosis is confirmed by aspiration and culture
  - *Dislocation*: 1–4% rate in the early postoperative period, decreases thereafter but does not go to zero; acute onset of pain with dislocation; radiographs are diagnostic
  - *Dissociation*: any part of either prosthesis can come apart; careful scrutiny of radiographs is necessary to identify incongruous components; dissociation of the head from the stem is obvious, dissociation of the plastic liner from the metal shell, less so
  - *Periprosthetic fracture*: may be present in patients with pain of sudden onset after trauma
  - *Loosening (septic or aseptic)*: aseptic loosening is gradual by history, with pain with weight bearing, start-up pain, and no rest pain

- **Essentials of Management**
  - Infection workup: WBC count, CRP, ESR, and aspiration
  - Dislocation: perform closed reduction or surgery
  - Surgery for periprosthetic fracture and septic joint

- **Pearl**

Relief of pain with local anesthetic injection into the hip joint suggests loosening if culture result is negative.

References

Biedermann R, et al.: Reducing the risk of dislocation after total hip arthroplasty: the effect of orientation of the acetabular component. J Bone Joint Surg Br 2005;87:762. [PMID: 15911655]

Helm CS, Greenwald AS: The rationale and performance of modularity in total hip arthroplasty. Orthopedics 2005;28:s1113. [PMID: 16190048]

Dislocation of the Total Hip Arthroplasty

ICD-9: 835

■ Essentials of Diagnosis

- Patient reports feeling that something "slipped out"; immediate pain, often excruciating, with instability of the hip
- Usually occurs shortly after total hip replacement surgery (within 3 mo), but can happen years later
- Position of the dislocated femoral head at time of radiographic examination may have nothing to do with mechanism of dislocation
- On physical exam, hip is usually in extension with internal rotation (posterior dislocation) or external rotation (anterior dislocation); affected leg is usually shorter
- Radiographic exam is diagnostic

■ Differential Diagnosis

- Periprosthetic femoral fracture
- Prosthetic component failure (fracture), femoral
- Prosthetic component failure (fracture or polyethylene dislocation), acetabular
- Acute infection

■ Treatment

- Closed reduction with conscious sedation is usually possible; in some cases, longitudinal traction with internal or external rotation under fluoroscopic control results in reduction; some posterior dislocations require reduction from the flexed, internally rotated position
- General anesthesia is sometimes necessary; occasionally open reduction is required; open reduction, if required, should be definitive in preventing further dislocations unless there is neural or vascular compromise, which requires urgent/emergent treatment
- An orthosis allowing motion in the "safe" range of motion is recommended

■ Pearl

Carefully check the sciatic and femoral nerves for function before attempting a closed reduction.

References

Peak EL, et al.: The role of patient restrictions in reducing the prevalence of early dislocation following total hip arthroplasty. A randomized, prospective study. J Bone Joint Surg Am 2005;87:247. [PMID: 15687143]

Soong M, et al.: Dislocation after total hip arthroplasty. J Am Acad Orthop Surg 2004;12:314. [PMID: 15469226]

Total Ankle Arthroplasty

ICD-9: not applicable

- ■ Essential Concepts
  - Generally performed for degenerative joint disease or rheumatoid arthritis; most convincing indication is ankle and subtalar arthritis in a patient with limited activity (avoids pantalar fusion)
  - Procedure is difficult due to limited soft tissue coverage (more infections) and large forces on small surface area of prosthetic support, leading to tibial hardware loosening and settling into softer bone laterally
  - Poor long-term results and failures led to arthrodesis as surgery of choice in 1980s
  - STAR and Buechel-Pappas prostheses are uncemented, with 3 components and mobile bearing (STAR has ~70% 5-y success rate); agility prosthesis is uncemented, 2-component, with a fixed-bearing design (a 9-y follow-up study reported 11% revision rate, and radiographically 19% subtalar arthritis, 15% talonavicular arthritis, and 8% syndesmosis nonunion)
  - Contraindications: infection, talus osteonecrosis, Charcot joints, extreme osteoporosis, severe arteriosclerosis
  - Possible contraindications: mental and neurologic disorders

- ■ Essentials of Management
  - Alternate treatment options: ankle fusion; ankle-foot orthosis
  - Agility prosthesis requires greater bone resection and arthrodesis of distal tibiofibular syndesmosis
  - With STAR and Buechel-Pappas prostheses, medial and lateral malleoli remain unresurfaced, resulting in less bone resection

- ■ Pearl

This procedure is barely out of the experimental stage and should be recommended to patients cautiously.

References

Anderson T, et al.: Uncemented STAR total ankle prostheses. J Bone Joint Surg Am 2004;86-A:103. [PMID: 15466751]

Gill LH: Challenges in total ankle arthroplasty. Foot Ankle Int 2004;25:195. [PMID: 15132926]

Hintermann B, Valderrabano V: Total ankle replacement. Foot Ankle Clin 2003;8:375. [PMID: 12911248]

Knecht SI, et al.: The agility total ankle arthroplasty. Seven to sixteen-year follow-up. J Bone Joint Surg Am 2004;86-A:1161. [PMID: 15173288]

Stengel D, et al.: Efficacy of total ankle replacement with meniscal-bearing devices: a systematic review and meta-analysis. Arch Orthop Trauma Surg 2005;125:109. [PMID: 15690167]

Total Shoulder Arthroplasty: Painful

ICD-9: V43.61 Shoulder arthroplasty; 996.66 Infected arthroplasty; 996.41 Aseptic loosening

- ■ Essential Concepts
  - • Indicated for patients with severe osteoarthritis (OA), rheumatoid arthritis (RA), post-traumatic arthritis, osteonecrosis, and dislocation arthropathy
  - • Contraindicated in patients with sepsis, rotator cuff tears, and nonfunctioning deltoids
  - • Because arthritis of the glenohumeral joint is much less common than that of the knee and hip, total shoulder arthroplasty (TSA) is performed much less frequently than arthroplasty of the knee and hip
  - • Pain relief after TSA is ~90–95%
  - • Complications include glenoid loosening (most common), instability or dislocation, late rotator cuff tears, periprosthetic fractures, infections, nerve injury (axillary nerve most common), and component dissociation

- ■ Essentials of Management
  - • Physical exam demonstrates a swollen, erythematous, painful shoulder in patients with infections
  - • Careful evaluation of muscle weakness and diminished sensation can help determine if a nerve injury is present
  - • Elevated WBC count, ESR, and CRP are nonspecific indicators of inflammation and suggestive of infection
  - • Joint aspiration under strict sterile technique can yield fluid that can help make the diagnosis; indications of probable infection are positive Gram stain, WBC count >50,000 and positive cultures
  - • Radiographs are essential in working up a painful TSA; plain radiographs can assist in diagnosing fractures, component loosening, and dislocation; an axillary view helps in diagnosing more subtle instabilities

- ■ Pearl

Typical results after a TSA yield range of motion that is between 50% and 80% of a normal glenohumeral joint. Commonly a patient with a TSA is only able to obtain 90 degrees of forward flexion.

Reference

Bryant D, et al.: A comparison of pain, strength, range of motion, and functional outcomes after hemiarthroplasty and total shoulder arthroplasty in patients with osteoarthritis of the shoulder. A systematic review and meta-analysis. J Bone Joint Surg Am 2005;87:1947. [PMID: 16140808]

Total Knee Arthroplasty: Painful

ICD-9: V43.65 Knee arthroplasty; 996.66 Infected arthroplasty; 996.77 Aseptic loosening

- **Essential Concepts**
  - Total knee arthroplasty is the surgical treatment of end-stage inflammatory or degenerative arthritis of the knee, performed by replacing articular surfaces of the tibia, femur, and usually patella; femoral component is metal, tibial is usually metal with a plastic-bearing surface insert, and patellar is usually plastic
  - Problems, and associated symptoms, include:
  - *Infection*: acute-onset or chronic pain, suspicious for infection with elevated CRP and ESR; WBC count may be normal and patient afebrile; wound may or may not be inflamed; diagnosis is confirmed by aspiration and culture
  - *Dissociation*: the tibial plastic-bearing surface can fracture, wear, or separate from the tibial baseplate; some designs allow motion of the plastic component; careful scrutiny of radiographs can occasionally discern whether this is the problem
  - *Instability*: can manifest at tibiofemoral or patellofemoral joint; after total replacement most knees have slight anterior laxity due to sacrifice of the anterior cruciate ligament, but mediolateral and posterior stability should be good in flexion and extension; history and physical exam can discern this instability; lateral radiographs may show anterior subluxation of the femur on the tibia; patellofemoral instability is manifested by pain, subluxation, and even dislocation; Merchant or sunrise radiographs aid diagnosis
  - *Loosening*: aseptic loosening is gradual by history, with pain on weight bearing and start-up, but not at rest
  - *Periprosthetic fracture*: may be present in patients with pain of sudden onset after trauma

- **Essentials of Management**
  - Infection workup: WBC, CRP, ESR, and aspiration
  - Dislocation: closed reduction versus surgery
  - Surgery for periprosthetic fracture and septic joint

- **Pearl**

The knee wound area may remain warm to the touch (normally) for up to 1 y.

References

Cuckler JM: The infected total knee: management options. J Arthroplasty 2005;20:33. [PMID: 15991126]

Gonzalez MH, Mekhail AO: The failed total knee arthroplasty. J Am Acad Orthop Surg 2004;12:436. [PMID: 15615509]

Periprosthetic Fractures of Hip, Knee, or Shoulder

ICD-9: 996.44

- ■ Essentials of Diagnosis
  - • Fracture can occur in the vicinity of an arthroplasty prosthesis
  - • Fracture can be immediately adjacent to the end of the prosthesis, around the prosthesis, involve a loose prosthesis, or an intraoperative fracture; fracture patterns are classified for each joint based on these factors
  - • Patients have pain, possibly instability, and swelling
  - • Radiographs define the problem (eg, loose prosthesis; displaced fracture; fracture above, at, or below the distal tip of the prosthesis)

- ■ Differential Diagnosis
  - • Loose prosthesis
  - • Dislocation of prosthesis
  - • Stress fracture
  - • Septic prosthetic joint

- ■ Treatment
  - • Depends on the location and quality of the bone
  - • Femoral hip periprosthetic fractures are either reduced and fixed with internal fixation or revised to a longer stem, using the stem as the internal splint
  - • Femoral knee periprosthetic fractures are treated with either reduction and fixation or, if bone quality is poor, with distal femoral replacement
  - • Tibial fractures can be treated with revision to a long stem; undisplaced fractures are frequently treated closed
  - • Humeral fractures that result in instability of the prosthesis require revision with a longer stem and possibly a plate; those that are stable often can be treated nonoperatively; short oblique fractures should be treated with early stable fixation

- ■ Pearl

Nonunions of proximal or distal periprosthetic fractures of the femur are rare but are difficult to manage.

References

Fink B, et al.: Periprosthetic fractures of the femur associated with hip arthroplasty. Arch Orthop Trauma Surg 2005;125:433. [PMID: 15999276]

Kim KI, et al.: Periprosthetic fractures after total knee arthroplasties. Clin Orthop 2006;446:167. [PMID: 1668003]

McDonnough EB, Crosby LA: Periprosthetic fractures of the humerus. Am J Orthop 2005;34:586. [PMID: 16450687]

Osteoarthritis of the Shoulder

ICD-9: 715.11

- ■ Essentials of Diagnosis
  - Osteoarthritis (OA) of the shoulder (glenohumeral arthritis) affects fewer US adults than OA of the hip or knee; it can be a result of cuff arthropathy, from chronic rotator cuff (RC) tear
  - Pain occurs in the shoulder area, accentuated by motion
  - History of limited use due to pain; night pain that interrupts sleep; internal rotation contracture; adduction contracture; occasionally crepitus on motion of the shoulder
  - AP radiographs show narrowing of the joint space, osteophyte formation, periarticular cysts, and subchondral sclerosis; the glenoid becomes biconcave because the humeral head rides on the posterior glenoid; the biconcave glenoid can be visualized on axillary radiographs or CT scan
  - Physical exam: OA of the shoulder can be difficult to distinguish from RC pathology; in OA patients have pain during glenohumeral rotation in both abduction and adduction; with RC pathology, pain occurs in abduction but often not in adduction

- ■ Differential Diagnosis
  - RC tear or impingement
  - Cervical disk disease
  - Rheumatoid arthritis
  - Osteonecrosis
  - Secondary OA: cuff arthropathy, post-traumatic

- ■ Treatment
  - NSAIDs plus acetaminophen for pain relief; glucosamine and chondroitin sulfate; activity modification; exercise for muscle strengthening
  - Corticosteroid injections for patients with moderate joint space narrowing, or to relieve pain and postpone surgery in severe arthritis
  - Surgical options: RC tear repair, total shoulder replacement, hemiarthroplasty replacement for irreparable RC tears; arthrodesis (fusion) for deltoid paralysis and heavy laborers

- ■ Pearl

RC competence can be tested by determining external rotation strength (infraspinatus) and internal rotation (subscapularis) with the arm at the side.

References

Iannotti JP, Kwon YW: Management of persistent shoulder pain: a treatment algorithm. Am J Orthop 2005;34:16. [PMID: 16450692]

Parsons IM, et al.: Glenohumeral arthritis and its management. Phys Med Rehabil Clin N Am 2004;15:447. [PMID: 15145425]

Osteoarthritis of the Ankle

ICD-9: 715.17

- ■ Essentials of Diagnosis
  - Primary osteoarthritis (OA) of the ankle is much less common than OA in the hip and knee
  - Trauma is the most common cause
  - Post-traumatic arthritis of the ankle occurs in ~14% of ankle injuries and is related to adequacy of articular reduction
  - Plain radiographs provide adequate imaging for diagnosis OA of the ankle with joint space narrowing

- ■ Differential Diagnosis
  - Ankle fracture
  - Osteochondritis dissecans
  - Ankle sprain
  - Subtalar osteoarthritis
  - Ankle instability

- ■ Treatment
  - In early stages, NSAIDS are the first line of treatment
  - Bracing can be helpful in alleviating pain and can be used to immobilize the ankle (lace-up brace, stirrup brace, ankle-foot orthosis)
  - Orthotics can be used to shift forces across the ankle joint to a more favorable distribution (medial or lateral heal wedges)
  - Injection with corticosteroids can be helpful
  - Once conservative treatments fail, surgical options can be considered (arthroscopic debridement, arthrodesis, and arthroplasty)
  - Arthroscopy has limited benefits in early arthritis
  - Arthrodesis in advanced arthritis of the ankle is considered the primary surgical treatment once all conservative measures have failed
  - Ankle arthroplasty is gaining acceptance as a treatment option, although it still is plagued by high failure and complication rates

- ■ Pearl

Because of the relatively smaller surface of the ankle compared with the hip and knee, the ankle joint carries loads twice as high as those other joints. Loads up to 5 times body weight occur during normal walking.

Reference

Thomas RH, Daniels TR: Ankle Arthritis. J Bone Joint Surg Am 2003;85:923. [PMID: 12728047]

Osteoarthritis of the Elbow

ICD-9: 715.12

- **Essentials of Diagnosis**
  - Osteoarthritis (OA) of the elbow is most common in men aged 20–60 y with a history of strenuous work, throwing sports, or trauma; prevalence is ~2% in the general population; male:female ratio is 4:1
  - Presenting symptoms: pain, stiffness, mechanical locking, and occasionally deformity
  - Physical exam: crepitus on range of motion (ROM), loss of ROM, swelling
  - Plain radiographs are diagnostic and demonstrate osteophytes, loose bodies, and joint space narrowing

- **Differential Diagnosis**
  - Elbow fractures
  - Elbow dislocations
  - Osteochondritis dissecans
  - Elbow instability
  - Synovial chondromatosis
  - Medial or lateral epicondylitis

- **Treatment**
  - Rest, NSAIDs, activity modification (changes in work or sports activities long term)
  - Corticosteroid injections are often effective in improving symptoms but should be administered judiciously
  - There is some evidence that viscosupplementation with hyaluronic acid injections may diminish symptoms
  - For patients who do not respond to conservative treatment, surgery can be considered
  - In ulnohumeral arthroplasty, the joint is debrided, the capsule is released, and osteophytes are removed; this surgery should be reserved for patients with pain at end ROM; it can be done either open or arthroscopically
  - Total elbow arthroplasty is rarely indicated in patients with OA, who typically work hard with their arms; an elbow replacement does not hold up well to strenuous activity

- **Pearl**

OA of the elbow typically begins on the lateral (radiocapitellar) aspect of the elbow joint, which sees the highest valgus stresses.

Reference

Gramstad GD, Galatz LM: Management of elbow osteoarthritis. J Bone Joint Surg Am 2006;88:421. [PMID: 16452758]

Osteoarthritis of the Hip

ICD-9: 715.15

■ Essentials of Diagnosis

- ~300,000 total hip replacements are performed each year for osteoarthritis (OA) of the hip
- Patients who develop early OA of the hip commonly have a congenital or developmental predisposition (ie, developmental dysplasia of the hip, slipped capital femoral epiphysis, or Legg-Calvé-Perthes disease)
- Pain is usually in the groin or side of the hip, very seldom in the buttock
- History of limited walking distance (1–4 blocks) due to pain, pain going up or down stairs, night pain that interrupts sleep, and pain with sitting, especially with hip flexed
- Physical exam frequently shows loss of internal rotation, flexion contracture, decreased flexion, and adduction contracture, and occasionally crepitus on motion of the hip
- AP radiographs of the pelvis show narrowing of the joint space of one or both hips, osteophyte formation, periarticular cysts, and subchondral sclerosis

■ Differential Diagnosis

- Lumbar disk disease
- Chondrocalcinosis
- Gouty arthritis
- Rheumatoid arthritis
- Osteonecrosis

■ Treatment

- NSAIDs plus acetaminophen for pain relief; glucosamine and chondroitin sulfate; non–weight-bearing exercise (eg, swimming); weight loss
- Corticosteroid injections for patients with moderate joint space narrowing, or to postpone surgery
- Surgical options: total hip replacement, surface replacement; osteotomy in young patients; indications for each procedure depend on age, status of hip, activity, and weight of patient

■ Pearl

An arthrogram with local anesthetic can differentiate whether pain is arising from the lumbar spine or the hip.

References

Silva M, et al.: The biomechanical results of total hip resurfacing arthroplasty. J Bone Joint Surg Am 2004;86-A:40. [PMID: 14711943]

Towheed TE, et al.: Acetaminophen for osteoarthritis. Cochrane Database Syst Rev 2006;CD004257. [PMID: 16437479]

Osteoarthritis of the Knee

ICD-9: 715.16

- ■ Essentials of Diagnosis
  - ~400,000 total knee replacements are performed each year for osteoarthritis (OA) of the knee; the medial compartment of the knee is most likely to require surgery
  - History of limited walking distance (1–4 blocks) due to pain, pain going up or down stairs, and night pain that interrupts sleep; minimal pain with sitting
  - Physical exam shows joint line tenderness to palpation (usually medial), patellofemoral crepitus, quadriceps weakness, flexion contracture, and decreased flexion; varus deformity is common; effusion occurs only with activity
  - Standing, flexed knee radiographs show narrowing of the joint space; other radiographic findings are subchondral sclerosis, periarticular cysts, and osteophytes

- ■ Differential Diagnosis
  - Chondrocalcinosis
  - Gouty arthritis
  - Rheumatoid arthritis
  - Osteonecrosis

- ■ Treatment
  - NSAIDs plus acetaminophen for pain relief; glucosamine and chondroitin sulfate; non–weight-bearing exercise (eg, swimming); weight loss; orthoses are a possibility, if effective in correcting deformity, but are not well tolerated; lateral wedges can help mild medial OA
  - Corticosteroid or viscosupplementation injections for patients with moderate joint space narrowing
  - Surgical options: total knee replacement, unicompartmental replacement (usually medial), metal spacer procedures for affected medial compartment, or osteotomy; indications for each procedure depend on patient age, activity, and weight, and status of knee compartments

- ■ Pearl

MRI is not useful in the diagnosis of OA of the knee. If standing radiographs are normal, MRI may be appropriate to evaluate the knee for causes of pain other than OA.

References

Shimada S, et al.: Effects of disease severity on response to lateral wedged shoe insole for medial compartment knee osteoarthritis. Arch Phys Med Rehabil 2006;87:1436. [PMID: 17084116]

Osteonecrosis

ICD-9: 733.40

- **Essentials of Diagnosis**
  - Also called *avascular necrosis* (AVN); 10,000–20,000 new cases each year in the US
  - Occurs most often in the femoral head, medial condyle of the femur, humeral head, capitellum, scaphoid, lunate, talus, and second metatarsal head
  - Can be traumatic (as in femoral neck fracture, humeral head fractures, hip dislocations) or associated with alcohol consumption, corticosteroid use, smoking, sickle cell, caisson disease, microscopic fat emboli, or focal clotting; most common etiology is idiopathic; multiple factors probably combine to cause AVN
  - May be detectable 6 mo after the insult that causes it but is not symptomatic until bone collapses due to inability to remodel routine microtrauma
  - Complaint of pain in the affected joint area leads to diagnosis
  - Radiographs may not be helpful early in the disease; later, fluffy calcification is seen in the bone with collapse of the subchondral plate; early diagnosis, before radiographic changes, is made by MRI, which is very sensitive

- **Differential Diagnosis**
  - Gaucher disease
  - Bone bruise

- **Treatment**
  - Two basic categories: joint arthroplasty for joints beyond the point of no return (symptomatic), and joint-sparing procedures to try to restore blood supply to the necrotic bone, usually by drilling a hole, sometimes with adjunctive treatment (eg, growth factors) to stimulate bone growth; joint-sparing procedures are reserved for asymptomatic or mildly symptomatic lesions

- **Pearl**

Idiopathic AVN of the hip can be found in patients in their 20s and older.

References

Assouline-Dayan Y, et al.: Pathogenesis and natural history of osteonecrosis. Semin Arthritis Rheum 2002;32:94. [PMID: 12430099]

Hungerford DS, Jones LC: Asymptomatic osteonecrosis: should it be treated? Clin Orthop Relat Res 2004;124. [PMID: 15577476]

Lafforgue P: Pathophysiology and natural history of avascular necrosis of bone. Joint Bone Spine 2006;73:500. [PMID: 16931094]

Arthrodesis

ICD-9: V45.4 Status postarthrodesis; 718.5 Ankylosis; 718.55 Hip; 718.56 Knee

- ■ Essential Concepts
  - • Arthrodesis (fusion) creates a bony union between bones of a diseased joint; ankylosis (fibrous union) may retain some motion
  - • Any joint can undergo arthrodesis; spontaneous ankylosis can occur after infection, trauma, or other disease process
  - • Can cause degeneration in adjacent joints and increased energy requirements of that extremity
  - • History of no motion at the joint, minimal if any pain, no pain with weight bearing in lower extremity fusions; usually a history of septic arthritis
  - • Physical exam shows no motion at the joint area; nontender to palpation if fully healed
  - • Radiographs show bridging of bone across the joint
  - • Arthrodesis can be performed surgically, most often to relieve pain of arthritis; indications include post-traumatic arthritis, rheumatoid arthritis, infection, neuromuscular conditions with instability of a joint, salvage of a failed total joint arthroplasty, and neuropathic joint (ie, Charcot joint)
  - • Bony surfaces in a surgical arthrodesis must be held motionless by internal or external fixation

- ■ Essentials of Management
  - • Surgical arthrodesis is most often performed in the ankle, knee, shoulder, hand, and hip; arthroscopic techniques can be employed for fusion of some joints; arthrodesis of the ankle results in long-term arthritic changes in the ipsilateral foot
  - • Arthrodesis of the hip and knee can be converted to total joint arthroplasty, if infection is clearly resolved

- ■ Pearl

Arthrodesis is a treatment of last resort in patients with infection of the hip, knee, shoulder, or ankle; shoulder arthrodesis is indicated in deltoid paralysis.

References

Coester LM, et al.: Long-term results following ankle arthrodesis for post-traumatic arthritis. J Bone Joint Surg Am 2001;83A:219. [PMID: 11216683]

Panagiotopoulos KP, et al.: Conversion of hip arthrodesis to total hip arthroplasty. Instr Course Lect 2001;50:297. [PMID: 11372328]

Stover MD, et al.: Hip arthrodesis: a procedure for the new millennium? Clin Orthop Relat Res 2004;(418):126. [PMID: 15043103]

Hip Labral Tear

ICD-9: 843.9

- **■ Essentials of Diagnosis**
  - The labrum is the cartilaginous extension of the bony acetabulum; it deepens the acetabulum to stabilize the hip
  - Two types of tears: traumatic (appear triangular on MRI) and degenerative (appear thick and rounded on MRI)
  - Patients have hip pain and mechanical symptoms (clicking, catching, locking)
  - Pain is referred to the hip (groin) with marked flexion and sometimes extension while the hip is held in internal or external rotation)
  - Radiographs are essentially normal, so a high index of suspicion is necessary; MRI arthrogram with contrast is the most sensitive imaging study
  - Injection of lidocaine is diagnostic if a tear is demonstrated and the pain is relieved

- **■ Differential Diagnosis**
  - Chondral lesion
  - Early degenerative joint disease
  - Iliopsoas bursitis or tendonitis
  - Osteonecrosis

- **■ Treatment**
  - If conservative treatment (activity modification and NSAIDs) is ineffective, arthroscopic labral repair or excision is indicated

- **■ Pearl**

Labral tears have been shown to have a role in the development of degenerative joint disease of the hip.

References

McCarthy JC: The diagnosis and treatment of labral and chondral injuries. Instr Course Lect 2004;53:573. [PMID: 15116646]

McCarthy JC, et al.: The Otto E. Aufranc Award: the role of labral lesions to development of early degenerative hip disease. Clin Orthop 2001;393:25. [PMID: 11764355]

Infections

Acute Bursitis

ICD-9: 726; 726.33 Olecranon; 726.65 Prepatellar

- ■ Essentials of Diagnosis
  - • Two forms: septic (infectious) and nonseptic (inflammatory)
  - • Infectious: usually due to hematogenous spread; affects mainly olecranon bursa and prepatellar bursa
  - • Inflammatory: affects olecranon, prepatellar, trochanteric, sub-acromial, and retrocalcaneal bursae
  - • Nonseptic bursitis can be painless with swelling from fluid in the bursa and no signs of inflammation; crystal deposition disease can have the clinical appearance of a septic bursitis
  - • In septic (or gouty) bursitis, pain is severe but joint motion is limited only at extremes
  - • Bursa aspiration can be performed for diagnosis and treatment; use care to avoid entering the joint, which could then become infected; purulent material does not confirm diagnosis of sepsis
  - • In 18–48% of patients, aspiration cultures are negative; in only 50% of blood cultures are results positive
  - • Acutely painful to palpation
  - • Radiographs are not usually helpful in diagnosis

- ■ Differential Diagnosis
  - • Gout, pseudogout
  - • Rheumatoid arthritis
  - • Septic joint

- ■ Treatment
  - • For septic arthritis, aspiration prior to antibiotic therapy is the first step in treatment; nonseptic bursitis can be treated with aspiration and cortisone injection; definitive treatment for both forms, if unresponsive to conservative measures, is resection of the bursa; arthroscopic bursectomy is a possible treatment
  - • Splinting the joint in a stable position is usually performed

- ■ Pearl

Range of motion can be used to clinically differentiate bursitis from septic arthritis. In septic arthritis, any motion of the joint is painful, whereas in bursitis, the joint is only painful at extremes of motion (eg, pronation and supination are painful in a septic joint but not if the bursa alone is involved).

References

Ogilvie-Harris DJ, Gilbart M: Endoscopic bursal resection: the olecranon bursa and prepatellar bursa. Arthroscopy 2000;16:249. [PMID: 10750004]

Small LN, Ross JJ: Suppurative tenosynovitis and septic bursitis. Infect Dis Clin North Am 2005;19:991. [PMID: 16297744]

Cellulitis

ICD-9: 682.9

- **Essentials of Diagnosis**
  - Infection of the skin or subcutaneous tissues by group A streptococci (most common) or *Staphylococcus aureus*
  - Patients have progressively worsening pain, swelling, erythema, and warmth; no abscess formation
  - Fever, elevated WBC count, lymphangitis, and lymphadenopathy are present
  - Radiographs, ultrasound, and MRI can aid in diagnosis

- **Differential Diagnosis**
  - Thrombophlebitis
  - Osteomyelitis
  - Septic arthritis
  - Necrotizing fasciitis
  - Myositis
  - Tinea corpus
  - Charcot joint
  - Stasis dermatitis
  - Contact dermatitis

- **Treatment**
  - Culture-sensitive antibiotics, initially penicillinase-resistant penicillin; blood cultures are not routinely useful for such infections
  - Alternative antibiotics: erythromycin, first-generation cephalosporins, amoxicillin-clavulanate, azithromycin, and clarithromycin
  - Antibiotic therapy may isolate the infection into an abscess; ultrasound and CT can be helpful in diagnosis of abscess, allowing surgical or interventional radiology drainage

- **Pearl**

The signs of inflammation—rubor, calor, tumor, dolor—are signs of inflammation, *not infection. Venous stasis (eg, especially around an extremity wound) can cause redness, warmth, and swelling. However, infection (bacteria) must be present for diagnosis of cellulitis.*

References

Falagas ME, Vergidis PI: Narrative review: diseases that masquerade as infectious cellulitis. Ann Intern Med 2005;142:47. [PMID: 15630108]

Stevenson A, et al.: The utility of blood cultures in the management of non-facial cellulitis appears to be low. N Z Med J 2005;118:U1351. [PMID: 15778752]

Acute Septic Arthritis

ICD-9: 711.0

- Essentials of Diagnosis
  - Usually due to hematogenous spread of bacteria; knee, hip, ankle, shoulder, and wrist joints are most often affected (in that order)
  - Most common in adults, but most serious sequelae from infection occur in children (destruction of physis)
  - Immunocompromised states and systemic illnesses (diabetes, alcoholism, cirrhosis, HIV) increase the risk for septic joints
  - Enzymatic degradation of joints can begin as early as 8 h after inoculation; *Staphylococcus aureus* is particularly aggressive in degrading articular cartilage
  - Pain is acute, with marked pain on motion of the joint
  - Joint aspiration usually shows WBC count >50,000, but much lower counts can be found if the joint is aspirated early in the disease process; a PMN count >75% of the total count is strongly suggestive of infection; low glucose level (<0.5 of the blood value) in the joint is also suggestive of infection
  - WBC count >100,000 is nearly diagnostic of septic arthritis and most often requires surgical debridement
  - In 18–48% of patients, aspiration cultures are negative; in only 50% of blood cultures are results positive
  - Radiographs are not usually helpful in diagnosis

- Differential Diagnosis
  - Gout, pseudogout
  - Rheumatoid arthritis
  - Charcot joint
  - Synovitis of the hip (in children)

- Treatment
  - Aspiration prior to antibiotic therapy is the first step; early drainage (arthroscopic, surgical) is important to prevent damage to cartilaginous structures (especially in children)
  - Splint joint in a stable position and monitor after aspiration and antibiotic use to determine efficacy of treatment

- Pearl

Gonorrhea is the most likely pathogen in young, sexually active patients and may be treated with antibiotics rather than surgical drainage.

Reference

Smith JW, et al.: Infectious arthritis: clinical features, laboratory findings and treatment. Clin Microbiol Infect 2006;12:309. [PMID: 16524406]

Acute Osteomyelitis

ICD-9: 730.2

- ■ Essentials of Diagnosis
  - Bone and bone marrow infection that is most commonly due to hematogenous spread in children; *Staphylococcus aureus* causes most cases
  - Frequently occurs after upper respiratory infection or incompletely treated distant infection; can occur from direct inoculation of an open fracture
  - Hematogenous form usually occurs in the metaphysis
  - Acute pain is caused by the pressure of pus under the periosteum
  - Early, in small children, the pain may be poorly localized, resulting in only a limp extremity or reluctance to bear weight
  - Fever and leukocytosis are usually, but not always, present; ESR and CRP are elevated
  - Obtain blood cultures and aspiration of bone for culture
  - Plain radiographs are not helpful for 10–14 days, when bone lysis, osteopenia, necrosis, and periosteal elevation appear
  - MRI with gadolinium may be helpful

- ■ Differential Diagnosis
  - Fracture
  - Septic joint
  - Toxic synovitis
  - Juvenile rheumatoid arthritis
  - Tumors

- ■ Treatment
  - Administer IV antibiotics; indications for operative intervention are abscess drainage, debridement of infected tissues, and refractory cases that are not responding to antibiotics
  - Long-term follow-up is necessary to diagnose and treat angular deformities and limb-length inequalities

- ■ Pearl

Reluctance of a child to walk or bear weight on a leg may be due to osteomyelitis of the spine. A bone scan can localize lesions for MRI evaluation.

Reference

McCarthy JJ, et al.: Musculoskeletal infections in children: basic treatment principles and recent advancements. Instr Course Lect 2005;54:515. [PMID: 15948476]

Osteomyelitis Due to Open Fractures

ICD-9: 730.0 Acute; 730.1 Chronic

- Essentials of Diagnosis
  - Can present acutely or chronically
  - Early infection, secondary to gross contamination of wound, can be diagnosed in a nonhealing wound or by wound breakdown and drainage after an open fracture
  - Late, chronic osteomyelitis is diagnosed by chronic, sometimes intermittent, drainage from the fracture area for months or years
  - Early infection sometimes clears after the fracture is healed and foreign bodies (plates, rods) are removed
  - Elevated ESR, CRP, and WBC count, if the wound is not draining
  - Plain radiographs can be diagnostic
  - Bone scan or MRI (with gadolinium) has more sensitivity; MRI shows edema in the bone, which is very suggestive of osteomyelitis
  - CT scan can show sequestra—pieces of dead bone that are a nidus for the infection
  - Indium WBC scan may not be helpful unless chronic osteomyelitis has an acute component

- Differential Diagnosis
  - Soft tissue or surgical site infection (not involving bone)
  - Septic joint
  - Neoplasm

- Treatment
  - Perform extensive debridement to remove all devitalized tissue; eliminate dead space by soft tissue coverage, antibiotic beads, or both; restore blood supply with free flaps where indicated
  - Remove foreign bodies such as fracture fixation devices when fracture stability can be maintained without them, or by using other fixation
  - Ilizarov bone transport may be necessary after extensive bone debridement
  - Culture-directed IV antibiotics, sometimes in combinations to avoid resistance

- Pearl

Chronic, draining, osteomyelitis is not an emergency. The drainage indicates that the wound is decompressed and the patient is not septic.

Reference

Calhoun JH, Manring MM: Adult osteomyelitis. Infect Dis Clin North Am 2005;19:765. [PMID: 16297731]

Osteomyelitis of the Spine

ICD-9: 730.00 Acute; 730.10 Chronic

■ Essentials of Diagnosis

- Osteomyelitis of the spine comprises about 1% of pyogenic skeletal infections but may have severe neurologic ramifications
- May be hematogenous or a result of surgical intervention
- S*taphylococcus aureus* is the most common pathogen
- Teenagers, older patients, debilitated patients, diabetics, and IV drug users are most at risk
- History of acute spinal pain with tenderness and spasm at the affected level; fever in nearly 50% of patients, muscle spasm in 90%, weight loss
- Neurologic deficit may be present or may develop
- ESR and CRP are elevated
- Plain films may show osteopenia, soft tissue swelling (loss of psoas shadow), and disk narrowing initially, followed by endplate destruction
- MRI is the best modality to differentiate from tumor; infections affect both the vertebral body and disk space, whereas tumors usually affect only the vertebral body
- Bone scan shows increased uptake at the affected level

■ Differential Diagnosis

- Pott disease (affects adjacent vertebral bodies and skips the disks)
- Neoplasm
- Fungal osteomyelitis of the spine

■ Treatment

- Antibiotics may be sufficient, combined with spinal immobilization
- Decompression with or without strut graft for neurologic deficit or with epidural abscess formation

■ Pearl

Juvenile diskitis is more common than juvenile osteomyelitis of the spine.

Reference

Tay, BK, et al.: Spinal infections. J Am Acad Orthop Surg 2002;10:188. [PMID: 12041940]

Tuberculosis of the Spine (Pott Disease)

ICD-9: 015.0

- **Essentials of Diagnosis**
  - Tubercular osteomyelitis of the spine is common in immigrants from less-developed countries; the indolent nature of tuberculosis leads to slow progression to kyphosis and severe neurologic ramifications
  - May spread hematogenously through the arterial system from another organ
  - Neurologic deficit may be present or may develop
  - History of indolent, chronic spinal pain at any level
  - Kyphosis is usually apparent on physical exam
  - Infection is often present in the thoracic spine or at the thoracolumbar junction, and usually involves several levels; disk spaces are spared
  - Plain films may show osteopenia, soft tissue swelling (loss of psoas shadow), vertebral body destruction, and kyphosis, with disk preservation
  - Bone scan shows a destructive process
  - MRI is the best modality to differentiate from tumor

- **Differential Diagnosis**
  - Fungal osteomyelitis of the spine
  - Neoplasm (metastatic [more common] or primary tumor)

- **Treatment**
  - Antibiotics specific to culture results
  - Anterior debridement and decompression with or without posterior instrumentation for advanced cases; more limited approaches for less severe cases or sicker patients

- **Pearl**

The diagnostic clue to the presence of tuberculosis is that the disk is preserved, whereas in bacterial osteomyelitis of the spine, the disk is destroyed.

References

Gasbarrini AL, et al.: Clinical features, diagnostic and therapeutic approaches to haematogenous vertebral osteomyelitis. Eur Rev Med Pharmacol Sci 2005;9:53. [PMID: 15852519]

Swanson AN, et al.: Chronic infections of the spine: surgical indications and treatments. Clin Orthop Relat Res 2006;444:100. [PMID: 16523133]

Atypical Infection of the Hand

ICD-9: 015.5 Tuberculosis; 031.9 Atypical mycobacteria;
117 Mycoses

- **Essentials of Diagnosis**
  - Causative organisms: *Mycobacterium marinum, kansasii, avium, bovis, intracellulare; Coccidioides immitis; Histoplasma capsulatum; Blastomyces dermatitidis*
  - Usually occurs in patients aged 50–80 y, in the distal upper extremity
  - May occur after puncture wound about 6 wk before onset of symptoms; *M marinum* should be suspected in seacoast environment or fishtank exposure; soil contact should suggest fungal infection
  - Patients are often immunocompromised (eg, diabetic, receiving anti—tumor necrosis factor therapy)
  - Presenting symptom is tenosynovitis or simply a soft tissue mass; no systemic symptoms; affected area is frequently inflamed but not as tender as expected for size and redness
  - Roentgenographic evaluation is negative unless the bone is involved

- **Differential Diagnosis**
  - Primary neoplasm
  - Foreign body reaction
  - Osteomyelitis

- **Treatment**
  - Surgical intervention for debridement or synovectomy and culture combined with a medical regimen is usually successful
  - Long-term antibiotic or antifungal therapy may be necessary

- **Pearl**

A hand mass that looks infectious but is less symptomatic than would be expected should suggest a granulomatous infectious process. Diagnosis is frequently delayed due to failure to consider mycobacterial and fungal infections.

References

Aubry A, et al : Sixty-three cases of Mycobacterium marinum infection: clinical features, treatment, and antibiotic susceptibility of causative isolates. Arch Intern Med 2002;162:1746. [PMID: 12153378]

Bhatty MA, et al.: Mycobacterium marinum hand infection: case reports and review of the literature. Br J Plast Surg 2000;53:161. [PMID: 10878841]

Granulomatous Infection of Bone or Joint: Tuberculous or Fungal

ICD-9: 015.5 Tuberculosis; 031.9 Atypical mycobacteria; 112, 114–117 Mycoses; 711.4 Arthropathy; 730.8 Osteomyelitis

■ Essentials of Diagnosis

- Causative organisms: *Mycobacterium tuberculosis*, atypical mycobacteria, *Coccidioides immitis*, *Candida*
- 1% of coccidioidomycosis cases result in hematogenous spread, disseminated disease (20% are to bone and joints); *Candida* usually seeds hematogenously to intervertebral disks and knees
- 35% of extrapulmonary tuberculosis (TB) occurs in bone and joint (spine [50%], hip) from undetected pulmonary source
- Patients are often immunocompromised (eg, diabetic, receiving anti–tumor necrosis factor therapy)
- Symptoms often occur months after fungemia or surgery; usually indolent local pain, gradually increasing in severity
- Perform a PPD skin test in patients with chronic atypical musculoskeletal infections
- Radiographs show lysis, some reactive sclerosis in bony lesions, joint space narrowing, and irregular erosions; both sides of the joint are affected

■ Differential Diagnosis

- Osteomyelitis
- Neoplasm (primary or metastatic disease)
- Sarcoidosis
- Lymphoma
- Foreign body reaction

■ Treatment

- TB: Medical regimen is the same as for pulmonary TB; atypical mycobacterial and fungal infections are treated per culture results; long courses of antibiotics or antifungals often are required
- Surgical intervention (joint or spinal fusion) is sometimes necessary

■ Pearl

Granulomatous infectious disease should be part of the differential diagnosis for any lesion in bone. In endemic areas, consider coccidioidomycosis in a patient with a recent history of a febrile month-long respiratory problem.

References

Crum-Cianflone NF, et al.: Unusual presentations of coccidioidomycosis: a case series and review of the literature. Medicine (Baltimore) 2006;85:263. [PMID: 16974211]
Gardam M, Lim S: Mycobacterial osteomyelitis and arthritis. Infect Dis Clin North Am 2005;19:819. [PMID: 16297734]

7

Foot Problems

Anterior Tibial Tendon Rupture

ICD-9: 726.74

- Essentials of Diagnosis
  - Tendon can rupture at insertion into the surface of the medial cuneiform or beneath the superomedial limb of the inferior extensor retinaculum (usually the distal 3 cm of the tendon)
  - Rupture is degenerative, subtle, and chronic (acute is rare)
  - History of foot flap or toe catching on ground with walking
  - Pain over the anterior aspect of the ankle
  - Weakness of dorsiflexion of the foot (toe extensors are used to compensate for the tibialis anterior)
  - Occasionally a palpable mass is present on the anterior ankle
  - MRI is diagnostic if physical exam is equivocal

- Differential Diagnosis
  - Tenosynovitis
  - Stress fracture
  - Lumbar radiculopathy
  - Degenerative joint disease of the midtarsal joints
  - Neuroma of the dorsal midfoot

- Treatment
  - Determined by patient's symptoms and degree of impairment; older, less active patients can be treated conservatively using an ankle-foot orthosis with 90-degree downstop for 3–4 mo
  - Surgical repair is indicated in active, athletic patients; attach the tendon to the navicular or use a tendon graft if the tendon is too short to reach the cuneiform
  - Crutches for 1 wk and weight bearing as tolerated in a short-leg walking cast for 4–6 wk

- Pearl

Untreated, rupture may lead to pes planus and claw toes.

Reference

Anagnostakos K, et al.: Rupture of the anterior tibial tendon: three clinical cases, anatomical study, and literature review. Foot Ankle Int 2006;27:330. [PMID: 16701053]

Ankle Ligamentous Injuries

ICD-9: 845.02 Calcaneofibular; 845.01 Deltoid;
845.03 Distal tibiofibular (Syndesmotic)

- **Essentials of Diagnosis**

  - Most common musculoskeletal injury; lateral collateral ligament complex (anterior and posterior talofibular ligaments [ATFL, PTFL] and calcaneal fibular ligament [CFL]) is most often injured; medially, deltoid ligament can be injured as well as syndesmosis that tethers fibula to tibia
  - Injured ligaments are tender to palpation; laxity may be present, depending on the severity of the injury
  - For ankle ligament instability: perform both clinical and radiographic stress exams to further delineate the injury
  - Anterior drawer test with ankle at 30 degrees of plantar flexion and slight internal rotation tests ATFL; inversion stress on heel with ankle in dorsiflexion tests CFL
  - Syndesmotic injury: assess by palpation, presence of swelling >2 cm above ankle joint, presence of tenderness elicited by squeezing fibula and tibia together, pain above ankle with external rotation of ankle
  - MRI may be of some benefit in patients with equivocal exams
  - Patients with talonavicular and calcaneonavicular coalition often have a history of recurrent ankle sprains

- **Differential Diagnosis**

  - Fracture
  - Osteochondral injury
  - Peroneal tendon injury

- **Treatment**

  - Soft ankle brace, ice, and elevation are beneficial for all injuries; continue bracing from 1–4 mo, depending on severity of injury; acetaminophen or NSAIDs for analgesia

- **Pearl**

Syndesmotic disruptions with widening of the ankle mortise require surgical repair; chronic instability may also benefit from surgical reconstruction.

References

Petrella R, et al.: Efficacy of celecoxib, a cox-2-specific inhibitor, and naproxen in the management of acute ankle sprain: results of a double-blind, randomized controlled trial. Clin J Sport Med 2004;14:225. [PMID: 15273528]

van Os AG, et al.: Comparison of conventional treatment and supervised rehabilitation for treatment of acute lateral ankle sprains: a systematic review of the literature. J Orthop Sports Phys Ther 2005;35:95. [PMID 15773567]

Achilles Tendon Rupture

ICD-9: 727.67

- ■ Essentials of Diagnosis
  - Usually seen in 30–50-y-old "weekend warriors" secondary to eccentric contraction of the gastrocnemius-soleus complex
  - Ruptures usually occur 3–6 cm proximal to the insertion on the calcaneus because blood supply there is poorest
  - Patient complains of sudden pain and often a "pop" after a push-off movement; history may be negative for pain before rupture
  - Thompson test (squeezing calf with patient prone and knee flexed to 90 degrees) is positive (no motion at ankle) with a complete rupture, and patient cannot do a heel raise on the affected side
  - Patient is able to dorsiflex at the ankle because of intact flexors of the toes
  - Palpable defect and swelling is present a few centimeters above the heel
  - Primary care physicians missed 23% of ruptures in one study
  - MRI and ultrasonography can be helpful in diagnosing recurrent or partial ruptures but should not be necessary with complete rupture

- ■ Differential Diagnosis
  - Partial ruptures of the tendon
  - Tendonitis (inflammation of the tendon)
  - Tendinosis (degeneration of the tendon)

- ■ Treatment
  - Surgical treatment (end-to-end apposition) is preferred in younger patients, older active patients, and patients with ruptures that occurred >2 wk prior to visit
  - Chronic ruptures may require a V-Y-plasty, or surgical reconstruction with a flexor hallucis longus transfer
  - Nonsurgical treatment with serial casting in plantar flexion is an option in less active patients or poor surgical candidates

- ■ Pearl

Surgical treatment has a lower rate of rerupture than nonsurgical treatment.

References

Jarvinen TA, et al.: Achilles tendon disorders: etiology and epidemiology. Foot Ankle Clin 2005;10:255. [PMID: 15922917]

Khan RJ, et al.: Treatment of acute achilles tendon ruptures. A meta-analysis of randomized, controlled trials. J Bone Joint Surg Am 2005;87:2202. [PMID: 16203884]

Acquired Flatfoot Deformity

ICD-9: 734

- **Essentials of Diagnosis**
  - By definition, a patient with acquired flatfoot deformity at one time had a normal functioning longitudinal arch
  - Four main causes: posterior tibial tendon (PTT) dysfunction (rupture), arthrosis of the tarsometatarsal joint, Charcot changes in the midfoot, and talonavicular collapse
  - Deformities may include dorsal subluxation of the talonavicular or tarsometatarsal joint, valgus deformity of the rearfoot, or abduction of the forefoot
  - When the patient stands on toes, the calcaneus is in valgus rather than the normal inversion
  - PTT rupture is manifested by tenderness and swelling on palpation of the tendon sheath; PTT dysfunction, by weak inversion
  - Radiographs usually differentiate the cause

- **Differential Diagnosis**
  - PTT rupture
  - Tarsometatarsal arthrosis (Lisfranc fracture, 50%; primary arthrosis, 50%)
  - Talonavicular collapse (50% of patients with rheumatoid arthritis)
  - Charcot foot

- **Treatment**
  - Conservative management includes support of the longitudinal arch by using an ankle-foot orthosis
  - Surgical correction of posterior tibial tendon rupture includes reconstruction with flexor digitorum longus and calcaneal osteotomy if significant valgus hindfoot is present
  - Arthrodesis can be performed for problems with the talonavicular and tarsometatarsal joints

- **Pearl**

When the patient's foot is viewed from behind, more toes will be visible laterally on the affected side ("too many toes" sign).

References

Mankey MG: A classification of severity with an analysis of causative problem related to the type of treatment. Foot Ankle Clin 2003;8:461. [PMID: 14560899]

Pedowitz WJ, Kovatis P: Flatfoot in the adult. J Am Acad Orthop Surg 1995;3:293. [PMID: 10790667]

Peroneal Tendon Tears

ICD-9: 727.68

■ Essentials of Diagnosis

- Usually attritional, from mechanical irritation
- Isolated tears of either tendon are rare
- Peroneus brevis is more commonly torn than peroneus longus
- Tear may be acute (or acute on chronic); if so, patient may have a history of stress to ankle
- Palpation may demonstrate tenderness and swelling along the course of the tendon
- Weakness and pain in eversion may be evident
- MRI is the imagining modality of choice

■ Differential Diagnosis

- Lateral ankle sprain
- Proximal fifth metatarsal fracture
- Anterior process of calcaneus fracture
- Peroneal tendonitis
- Peroneal tendon subluxation
- Osteochondral injury of the ankle
- S1 radiculopathy

■ Treatment

- Immobilization is successful in 20% of cases; operative repair is needed in 80%

■ Pearl

Peroneal tendon tears can be a source of chronic lateral ankle pain.

References

Dombek MF, et al.: Peroneal tendon tears: a retrospective review. J Foot Ankle Surg 2003;42:250. [PMID: 14566716]

Wind WM, Rohrbacher BJ: Peroneus longus and brevis rupture in a collegiate athlete. Foot Ankle Int 2001;22:140. [PMID: 11249224]

Peroneal Tendonitis

ICD-9: 726.79

- **Essentials of Diagnosis**
  - Caused by trauma, repetitive motion activities (most common), or inflammatory arthropathies
  - Can lead to a cavus deformity as the peroneals weaken
  - Usually occurs behind the lateral malleolus as the peroneus longus pushes on the brevis
  - Common complaint is lateral ankle pain, worsened by activity, improved with rest and NSAIDs
  - Tenderness to palpation along peroneal tendons
  - Swelling along peroneal tendons
  - Pain with resisted eversion of the foot
  - MRI is diagnostic

- **Differential Diagnosis**
  - Peroneal tendon rupture
  - Chronic ankle sprain
  - Stress fracture of fifth metatarsal
  - Peroneal tendon subluxation
  - S1 radiculopathy

- **Treatment**
  - Immobilization in a cast for 4–6 wk for severe cases; milder cases can be treated with an ankle orthosis, activity modification, and NSAIDs
  - Surgical debridement if conservative measures fail

- **Pearl**

Consider peroneal tendonitis as a cause of lateral ankle pain in the patient with a previously fractured calcaneus.

References

Kijowski R, et al.: Magnetic resonance imaging findings in patients with peroneal tendinopathy and peroneal tenosynovitis. Skeletal Radiol 2007;36:105. [PMID: 17136379]

Leppilahti J, et al.: Longitudinal split of peroneus brevis tendon. A report on two cases. Ann Chir Gynaecol 2000;89:61. [PMID: 10791647]

Peroneal Tendon Subluxation & Dislocation

ICD-9: 726.79

■ Essentials of Diagnosis

- Caused by strong contraction of the peroneal tendons, combined with dorsiflexion of the ankle; this results in damage to the peroneal retinaculum, which holds the tendons in place
- Tendons subluxate anteriorly around the edge of the fibula with contraction and dorsiflexion, then are felt to pop out and return
- Usually acute but can be associated with recurrent ankle sprains
- Tenderness is posterior to the lateral malleolus
- Tendon may sublux when the foot is dorsiflexed
- Radiographs may show a small piece of bone lateral to the fibula
- MRI may be useful

■ Differential Diagnosis

- Ankle sprain (acute or chronic)
- Ankle instability
- Peroneal tendonitis
- Peroneal tendon tear or split

■ Treatment

- Immobilize in a splint in plantar flexion and inversion for acute injuries (failure rate ~50%)
- Acute surgical repair of the retinaculum is indicated in young, active patients and in less active patients who do not respond to nonoperative treatments
- If a shallow posterior fibular groove is noted at the time of retinacular repair, the groove is deepened to prevent recurrence

■ Pearl

Unlike patients with sprains, those with subluxations and dislocation often cannot recall exactly when the injury occurred.

References

Alanen J, et al.: Peroneal tendon injuries. Report of thirty-eight operated cases. Ann Chir Gynaecol 2001;90:43. [PMID: 11336369]

Ferran NA, et al.: Recurrent subluxation of the peroneal tendons. Sports Med 2006;36:839. [PMID: 17004847]

Tarsal Tunnel Syndrome

ICD-9: 355.5

- **Essentials of Diagnosis**

  - Compression or traction neuropathy of the posterior tibial nerve (or its branches, the medial or lateral plantar nerve) passing under the flexor retinaculum behind the medial malleolus
  - Symptoms: vague dysesthesias (burning) on plantar foot; aggravated by activity, relieved by rest, worst at night
  - Arterial vascular leash and scarring are the most common causes; other causes include lipoma, ganglion cyst, edema, and tumor in the tarsal tunnel
  - Tinel sign is present
  - NCS can be helpful in diagnosis
  - MRI is helpful to visualize space-occupying lesions

- **Differential Diagnosis**

  - Heel pain
  - Plantar fasciitis
  - Achilles tendonitis
  - Calcaneal stress fractures
  - Osteomyelitis
  - Posterior tibial tendon dysfunction

- **Treatment**

  - NSAIDs; ankle-foot orthosis in neutral inversion and eversion; steroid injection is usually 75% effective in relieving symptoms
  - Surgical release and nerve exploration yields 85% relief objectively and 51% relief subjectively

- **Pearl**

Rarely, the anomalous flexor digitorum accessorius longus may be the cause.

References

Bracilovic A, et al.: Effect of foot and ankle position on tarsal tunnel compartment volume. Foot Ankle Int 2006;27:431. [PMID: 16764800]

Burks JB, DeHeer PA: Tarsal tunnel syndrome secondary to an accessory muscle: a case report. J Foot Ankle Surg 2001;40:401. [PMID: 11777236]

Gondring WH, et al.: An outcomes analysis of surgical treatment of tarsal tunnel syndrome. Foot Ankle Int 2003;24:545. [PMID: 12921360]

Sammarco VJ, Nichols R: Orthotic management for disorders of the hallux. Foot Ankle Clin 2005;10:191. [PMID: 15831266]

Cavus Foot

ICD-9: 736.73

- **Essentials of Diagnosis**

  - Excessive elevation of the longitudinal arch due to fixed plantar flexion of the forefoot (anterior form), calcaneus dorsiflexion deformity (posterior form), and combined
  - Forefoot pronation and adduction; hindfoot varus (variable)
  - Pain on walking, standing; calf muscle atrophy; claw toes
  - Coleman "lateral block" test evaluates hindfoot flexibility and pronation of the forefoot
  - Weight-bearing radiographs: metatarsals are excessively plantar flexed, midfoot elevated, hindfoot in varus position, plantar flexion of talus reduced
  - Consider EMG if foot was previously normal (two-thirds of patients have a neurologic disorder); MRI of spinal cord to rule out tumor, dysraphic lesions; CT scan of head to rule out occult hydrocephalus

- **Differential Diagnosis**

  - Asymmetric or unilateral deformity: cerebral palsy, diastematomyelia (spinal cord dysraphism), spinal cord tumor, tethered cord
  - Symmetric or bilateral deformity: idiopathic, Becker muscular dystrophy, cerebral palsy, congenital pes cavus, Charcot-Marie-Tooth syndrome, dystonia musculorum deformans (equinovarus), Friedreich ataxia, poliomyelitis, arthrogryposis, occult hydrocephalus

- **Treatment**

  - Nonoperative, for mild deformity: soft-soled shoe, extra-depth shoe for significant claw toes; ankle-foot orthosis for significant motor deficit
  - Operative, early deformity: soft tissue release, tendon transfer (plantar fascia release, claw toe release)
  - Operative, fixed deformity: calcaneal osteotomy, metatarsal osteotomy

- **Pearl**

Progression of the deformity over time suggests a worsening neurologic disorder.

References

Burns J, et al.: Effective orthotic therapy for the painful cavus foot: a randomized controlled trial. J Am Podiatr Med Assoc 2006;96:205. [PMID: 16707631]

Joseph TN, Myerson MS: Correction of multiplanar hindfoot deformity with osteotomy, arthrodesis, and internal fixation. Instr Course Lect 2005;54:269. [PMID: 15948455]

Charcot Foot

ICD-9: 713.5

- ■ Essentials of Diagnosis
  - Also termed *neuropathic*, *neurotrophic*, or *neuroarthropathic joint*; diabetes is by far the leading cause
  - Marked destruction of joint surfaces, collapse of joint spaces, often with dislocations of one or more joints (the "4 Ds": Destruction, Dislocation, Deformity, Debris)
  - Calcification or bony debris in periarticular soft tissues
  - Pain is minimal or considerably less than would be expected given the degree of destruction
  - Exam can demonstrate bone rubbing on bone with minimal discomfort
  - Ankle or foot is often red, warm, and swollen; must differentiate from cellulitis or osteomyelitis—MRI can be helpful; also, erythema in the Charcot foot is more pronounced when the foot is held low ("dependent rubor"), whereas the cellulitic foot is erythematous whether elevated or not

- ■ Differential Diagnosis
  - Cellulitis
  - Osteomyelitis
  - Abscess
  - Fracture

- ■ Treatment
  - Primary goal is to limit joint destruction and preserve normal bony anatomy to prevent soft tissue ulceration
  - Initial treatment in acute phase should be immobilization and elevation of the foot; later surgery focuses on removing bony prominences and creating a stable joint with fusions and osteotomies
  - Fusions can be difficult to obtain and may require long immobilizations

- ■ Pearl

The tarsometatarsal joints most often undergo Charcot changes, followed by the talonavicular and calcaneocuboid joints. The phalanges and subtalar joint are rarely involved.

References

Ledermann HP, Morrison WB: Differential diagnosis of pedal osteomyelitis and diabetic neuroarthropathy: MR imaging. Semin Musculoskelet Radiol 2005;9:272. [PMID: 16247726]

Trepman E, et al.: Current topics review: charcot neuroarthropathy of the foot and ankle. Foot Ankle Int 2005;26:46. [PMID: 15680119]

Hallux Valgus (Bunion)

ICD-9: 735.0

■ Essentials of Diagnosis

- Lateral deviation of the great toe (bunion) is the most common deformity of the metatarsophalangeal (MTP) joint; 10 times more common in women, due to poorly fitting footwear
- Pain and irritation at the MTP joint, especially medially
- Standing radiographs of feet confirm diagnosis and determine therapy; angle between great toe and metatarsal (hallux valgus angle) should be <15 degrees and angle between first and second metatarsals (intermetatarsal angle), <9 degrees

■ Differential Diagnosis

- Hallux rigidus

■ Treatment

- Conservative therapy: shoe modification to enlarge the toe box, padding to take pressure off calluses or sesamoids, or to fill the first web space; exercises and activity modification
- Operative therapy depends on pathologic findings (how much deformity, arthritis, etc), patient factors (eg, age, activity level), and surgeon preference
- Generally, initial treatment is directed at the angle between the first and second metatarsals; if excessive, either a proximal or distal procedure is performed to correct it; then attention is directed at obtaining an MTP joint that is congruent and oriented in the proper direction
- Many procedures and combinations of procedures have been described; Keller procedure (resection arthroplasty) is used mainly for older, arthritic patients; arthrodesis is used for younger patients with arthritis or as a salvage procedure

■ Pearl

There is very limited evidence to suggest that conservative treatment is any better than no treatment.

References

Ferrari J, et al.: Interventions for treating hallux valgus (abductovalgus) and bunions. Cochrane Database Syst Rev 2004;CD000964. [PMID: 14973960]

Marks RM: Arthrodesis of the first metatarsophalangeal joint. Instr Course Lect 2005;54:263. [PMID: 15948454]

Sammarco VJ, Nichols R: Orthotic management for disorders of the hallux. Foot Ankle Clin 2005;10:191. [PMID: 15831266]

Hallux Rigidus

ICD-9: 735.2

- **Essentials of Diagnosis**
  - Limitation of motion and pain at the metatarsophalangeal (MTP) joint of the great toe (MTP joint arthritis)
  - Affects younger adults (≥30 y)
  - May be due to unrecognized chondral injury or to previous ligamentous or capsular injury (ie, "turf toe")
  - Pain occurs with passive dorsiflexion and is worsened by physical activity
  - Pain with axial loading and flexion-extension
  - Radiographs show osteophyte formation on the dorsal, distal first metatarsal

- **Differential Diagnosis**
  - Hallux varus
  - Hallux valgus
  - Hallus extensus

- **Treatment**
  - Conservative treatment consists of NSAIDs, stiff-soled shoe, and cortisone injection
  - Operative treatment is usually preferred by more active patients and is used for those unresponsive to conservative therapy
  - Cheilectomy (excision of the dorsal bone of the first metatarsal) may be beneficial in patients with mild arthritis
  - Various arthroplasty procedures are possible for more severely arthritic joints, (Keller, prosthetic) but success is modest, due to high complication rates
  - Arthrodesis of the first MTP is predictable in pain relief and longevity; activity is only modestly restricted

- **Pearl**

Lifting the great toe away from the floor in a standing patient causes pain in hallux rigidus.

References

Gibson JN, Thomson CE: Arthrodesis or total replacement arthroplasty for hallux rigidus: a randomized controlled trial. Foot Ankle Int 2005;26:680. [PMID: 16174497]

Sammarco VJ, Nichols R: Orthotic management for disorders of the hallux. Foot Ankle Clin 2005;10:191. [PMID: 15831266]

Sesamoid Fracture of the Great Toe

ICD-9: 827.0 Closed; 827.1 Open

■ Essentials of Diagnosis

- History of trauma, or crushing injury, dislocation of the first metatar-sophalangeal (MTP) joint, or increase in activity or training
- Pain (especially with weight bearing) at MTP
- Swelling, ecchymoses; tender to palpation
- Radiographs may be helpful; MRI may show the acuity of the process and differentiate a bipartite sesamoid

■ Differential Diagnosis

- Soft tissue trauma (ligament, tendon, injury)
- Reduced first MTP dislocation
- Stress fracture of sesamoid
- Inflamed bipartite sesamoid

■ Treatment

- Undisplaced fractures: accommodative (hard-soled) footwear and activity modification are appropriate
- Displaced fractures: great toe may need to be immobilized in flexion
- Excision should be the last resort as it can lead to disabling arthritis

■ Pearl

An inflamed bipartite sesamoid is less tender when the great toe is plantar flexed (in contrast to fracture, which is tender in all positions).

References

Dedmond BT, et al.: The hallucal sesamoid complex. J Am Acad Orthop Surg 2006;14:745. [PMID: 17148622]

Mittlmeier T, Haar P: Sesamoid and toe fractures. Injury 2004;35(suppl 2):SB87. [PMID: 15315883]

Ingrown Toenail

ICD-9: 703.0

- **Essentials of Diagnosis**
  - Occurs distally at the level of the nail bed or hyponychium (medial or lateral nail groove)
  - Can result from poorly fitting shoes or improper trimming technique
  - Acute: pain, swelling, cellulitis
  - Chronic: purulent exudate, granulation tissue

- **Differential Diagnosis**
  - Soft tissue infection of the toe
  - Herpetic whitlow
  - Subungual exostosis
  - Osteomyelitis in diabetic or immunocompromised patients

- **Treatment**
  - Preventive therapy includes trimming the nail locally, education on proper nail trimming (the nail should be trimmed distal to the nail fold), and ensuring proper fit of shoes
  - Oral antibiotics with preventive care can alleviate the early ingrown nail
  - Chronic cases require excision of a few millimeters of medial or lateral nail, back to the nail matrix
  - For recurrent ingrown nails, the medial or lateral portion of the nail, including the nail matrix, can be surgically removed to prevent recurrence; phenol can be used on the germinal matrix to reduce recurrence
  - In some cases, with nail deformity, a terminal amputation of the distal portion of the phalanx with the entire nail bed is necessary (Syme amputation)

- **Pearl**

Resection of the medial or lateral portion of the nail (or nail bed) should be limited to the minimum necessary to avoid impingement of the nail on the soft tissue.

References

Rounding C, Bloomfield S: Surgical treatments for ingrowing toenails. Cochrane Database Syst Rev 2005;CD001541. [PMID: 15846620]

Shaath N, et al.: A prospective randomized comparison of the Zadik procedure and chemical ablation in the treatment of ingrown toenails. Foot Ankle Int 2005;26:401. [PMID: 15913526]

Hammer Toe Deformity

ICD-9: 735.3

■ Essentials of Diagnosis

- Abnormal flexion posture of the proximal interphalangeal (PIP) joint of one of the lesser toes
- Worsened by hyperextension of the metatarsophalangeal joint
- May be fixed or passively correctable
- Caused by long-standing use of inappropriate footwear
- Callus or ulceration over the PIP joint, or at the tip of the toe

■ Differential Diagnosis

- Claw toe
- Mallet toe

■ Treatment

- Conservative management consists of appropriate footwear
- Surgical treatment for the flexible deformity is transfer of the long flexor to both sides of the extensor hood; this converts it from a deforming force to a correcting force (Girdlestone transfer)
- Fixed deformities are treated with condylectomy of the distal end of the proximal phalanx (DuVries) or with PIP fusion

■ Pearl

Any bunion deformity may have to be resolved in order to make room for the corrected second toe.

References

Coughlin MJ: Lesser toe abnormalities. Instr Course Lect 2003;52:421. [PMID: 12690869]

Edwards WH, Beischer AD: Interphalangeal joint arthrodesis of the lesser toes. Foot Ankle Clin 2002;7:43. [PMID: 12380380]

Jones S, et al.: Re: Arthrodesis of the toe joints with an intramedullary cannulated screw for correction of hammertoe deformity. Foot Ankle Int 2005;26:1101. [PMID: 16390648]

O'Kane C, Kilmartin T: Review of proximal interphalangeal joint excisional arthroplasty for the correction of second hammer toe deformity in 100 cases. Foot Ankle Int 2005;26:320. [PMID: 15829216]

Mallet Toe Deformity

ICD-9: 735.8

- ■ Essentials of Diagnosis
  - Abnormal flexion posture of the distal interphalangeal (DIP) joint of one of the lesser toes; usually affects the second toe because it is longer
  - May be fixed or passively correctable
  - The flexible deformity can be identified by obtaining correction with ankle plantar flexion, which loosens the toe flexors
  - Caused by long-standing use of inappropriate footwear
  - Callus or ulceration over the DIP joint, or at the tip of the toe
  - Nail deformity may be present

- ■ Differential Diagnosis
  - Claw toe
  - Hammer toe

- ■ Treatment
  - Extra depth in toe box of shoe; padding
  - Surgical correction of flexible deformities requires release of the flexor digitorum longus tendon at the level of the PIP joint; fixed deformities are treated with resection of the distal portion of the middle phalanx and pinning

- ■ Pearl

The distal phalanx callus can break down, causing an ulcer in diabetic patients.

Reference

Coughlin MJ: Lesser toe abnormalities. Instr Course Lect 2003;52:421. [PMID: 12690869]

Claw Toe Deformity

ICD-9: 735.3

■ Essentials of Diagnosis

- Abnormal extension posture of the metatarsophalangeal (MTP) joint and flexion of interphalangeal (IP) joints of usually all of the lesser toes, and sometimes the great toe
- Typically occurs in younger patients; may be flexible or rigid
- Caused by an imbalance of the intrinsic and extrinsic muscles of the toes
- Callus over the dorsal PIP joint or the plantar aspect of the metatarsal head, or both
- History of metatarsalgia; possible history of tibial fracture with injury or contracture of the long toe extensors and flexors

■ Differential Diagnosis

- Volkmann ischemic contracture
- Mallet toe
- Rheumatoid arthritis
- Neuromuscular disorders (ie, spinal cord injury)
- Cavus foot

■ Treatment

- Conservative management: extra-depth footwear; for flexible mild deformities, padding just proximal to the metatarsal heads
- Surgical treatment: initially directed at the hindfoot for cavus feet with deformity; flexible deformity is treated with transfer of the long flexor to both sides of the extensor hood and a hammer toe correction, if necessary (converts flexor from a deforming force to a correcting force [Girdlestone transfer]); for fixed deformity, soft tissue release, proximal phalangeal condylectomy (DuVries), and pinning of the MTP joint may be necessary in addition to Girdlestone transfer; Jones procedure (transfer of extensor hallucis longus to the metatarsal head) and IP joint fusion may be necessary for the great toe

■ Pearl

Passive plantar flexion of the ankle will allow correction of flexible claw toe deformities, while rigid, fixed deformities will not correct.

References

Ozdolap S, et al.: Modified Girdlestone-Taylor procedure for claw toes in spinal cord injury. Spinal Cord 2006;44:787. [PMID: 16568140]

Steensma MR, et al.: Flexor hallucis longus tendon transfer for hallux claw toe deformity and vertical instability of the metatarsophalangeal joint. Foot Ankle Int 2006;27:689. [PMID: 17038279]

Corns: Hard & Soft

ICD-9: 700.0

- **Essentials of Diagnosis**
  - Keratotic lesions that form over bony prominences of lesser toes due to excessive pressure on the skin; also known as *clavus mollum* (soft) and *clavus durum* (hard)
  - Hard corns commonly occur over the dorsal and lateral aspects of the fifth toe or over the proximal interphalangeal (PIP) joints of the lesser toes
  - Soft corns form between the toes in the web space due to pressure from the bony prominence on the opposing toe (usually in the fourth web space of the fourth toe, due to pressure from bones of the fifth toe); they are soft because moisture results in maceration

- **Differential Diagnosis**
  - Diabetic ulcer
  - Claw toes

- **Treatment**
  - Treatment is directed at removing the pressure; use of wider shoes, padding to shift pressure to other areas, and shaving the lesion can help relieve discomfort
  - Surgical treatment requires removing the offending bony prominence (minor procedures that are quite effective)
  - Soft corns can also be treated by surgical syndactyly of the fourth and fifth toes; this removes the skin between the toes and excises the corn

- **Pearl**

Soft corns may result from malunions of toe fractures.

Reference

Mann RA, Mann JA: Keratotic disorders of the plantar skin. Instr Course Lect 2004;53:287. [PMID: 15116622]

Tailor's Bunion

ICD-9: 727.1

- Essentials of Diagnosis
  - Prominence of the fifth metatarsal head can be a cause of metatarsalgia; callus formation is on the plantar or lateral aspect of the fifth metatarsal head
  - Called *tailor's bunion* or *bunionette* after the position in which a tailor sits
  - May be caused by splaying of the foot with loss of the transverse arch of the forefoot

- Differential Diagnosis
  - Aging of the foot with loss of transverse arch
  - Rheumatoid arthritis
  - Post-traumatic malunion

- Treatment
  - Orthotic devices may be helpful if caused by excessive pronation of the talus; wearing a wide, soft, lace-up shoe with metatarsal support helps relieve symptoms in mild and early cases; shaving the callus temporarily reduces pain
  - Surgery to narrow the foot by removing associated bony prominences and correcting deformities is appropriate in severe cases; surgery restores the normal intermetatarsal angle between the fourth and fifth metatarsals

- Pearl

Surgical treatment may require correction of both the plantar and *lateral deformities to alleviate the problem.*

References

Ajis A, et al.: Tailor's bunion: a review. J Foot Ankle Surg 2005;44:236. [PMID: 15940605]

Vienne P, et al.: Modified Coughlin procedure for surgical treatment of symptomatic tailor's bunion: a prospective followup study of 33 consecutive operations. Foot Ankle Int 2006;27:573. [PMID: 16919208]

Morton Interdigital Neuroma

ICD-9: 355.6

- ■ Essentials of Diagnosis
  - Well-localized area of pain usually in either the second or more commonly the third digital interspace of the metatarsal heads
  - Pathoanatomy is related to the position of the digital nerve relative to the transverse metatarsal ligament
  - Pain is aggravated by ambulation and relieved by rest, and can also be exacerbated by a tight-fitting shoe
  - 10 times more common in women than in men, and more common in those who wear high-heeled shoes
  - Physical exam: pain (sometimes shooting) is elicited with firm palpation of the interspace; squeezing of the forefoot causes pain, and occasionally a click (ie, Mulder click) of the neuroma in the intermetatarsal space; sometimes a palpable mass in the interspace
  - Not a true neuroma, but a degeneration of nerve tissue related to repeated trauma

- ■ Differential Diagnosis
  - Interdigital cyst
  - Metatarsophalangeal joint disease (arthritis)
  - Metatarsal stress fracture

- ■ Treatment
  - Conservative measures include use of a wider shoe and avoidance of narrow high-heeled shoes; metatarsal pad; and steroid injection
  - Surgical resection of the involved nerve in patients who do not respond to conservative care

- ■ Pearl

Ultrasound in the hands of an experienced ultrasonographer is the imaging modality of choice to confirm diagnosis.

References

Hassouna H, Singh D: Morton's metatarsalgia: pathogenesis, aetiology and current management. Acta Orthop Belg 2005;71:646. [PMID: 16459852]

Thomson CE, et al.: Interventions for the treatment of Morton's neuroma. Cochrane Database Syst Rev 2004;CD003118. [PMID: 15266472]

Metatarsophalangeal Joint Subluxation & Dislocation

ICD-9: 838.05

- **Essentials of Diagnosis**

  - Subluxation and dislocation of the metatarsophalangeal joint is most commonly caused by hallux valgus pressing against the second toe, with attenuation of ligaments, possibly from a steroid injection
  - Deformity progresses over a period of 3–6 mo; the second toe may cross over the great toe
  - Pain is on the dorsal and plantar aspects, because the proximal phalanx is dorsal and the metatarsal joint is plantar
  - Joint alignment is evaluated by using a Lachman-type test on the proximal phalanx
  - Radiographic evaluation is diagnostic in most patients

- **Differential Diagnosis**

  - Hammer toe deformity
  - Rheumatoid arthritis
  - Trauma
  - Fracture

- **Treatment**

  - If subluxation is stable, conservative management is recommended; this includes properly fitted shoes and cortisone injections
  - Surgical treatment is only indicated if medical management has failed, shoe wear is difficult, or there is a gross deformity that is unstable
  - Girdlestone procedure is indicated in patients with subluxation
  - Metatarsal neck osteotomies are indicated in patients with dislocation
  - Reduction can be attempted in patients with traumatic dislocation of the metatarsophalangeal joint(s)

- **Pearl**

Successful treatment usually requires consideration of the entire forefoot, especially any hallux valgus deformity.

References

Mendicino RW, et al.: Predislocation syndrome: a review and retrospective analysis of eight patients. J Foot Ankle Surg 2001;40:214. [PMID: 11924682]

Myerson MS, Jung HG: The role of toe flexor-to-extensor transfer in correcting metatarsophalangeal joint instability of the second toe. Foot Ankle Int 2005;26:675. [PMID: 16174496]

Heel Pain, Posterior

ICD-9: 719.47

- **Essentials of Diagnosis**
  - Common cause is Achilles tendinosis (tendonitis) related to more degenerative conditions that occur either at the insertion of the Achilles or proximal to the insertion by several centimeters; associated with physical activity
  - Patients have localized pain on use of the gastrocnemius
  - Physical exam shows tenderness and warmth at the insertion of the Achilles (insertional) or at the tendon proximal to the insertion; this area may be thickened (noninsertional)
  - Radiographs may show a calcaneal spur or calcific deposit at the insertion of the tendon, but it is not an acute finding

- **Differential Diagnosis**
  - Avulsion of the musculotendinous junction of the gastrocnemius
  - Achilles tendon rupture
  - Haglund deformity with retrocalcaneal bursitis
  - Lumbar radiculopathy
  - Tarsal tunnel syndrome

- **Treatment**
  - Achilles tendinosis is treated with NSAIDs, stretching exercises (especially eccentric loading training), activity modification, and a heel lift
  - Surgery to debride a degenerative tendon and remove calcific deposits is indicated if the patient is unresponsive to nonsurgical measures for 9 mo
  - If Haglund deformity is present, it is also resected

- **Pearl**

Levofloxacin is the fluoroquinolone associated with the highest rate of tendinopathy.

References

Leone R, et al.: Adverse drug reactions related to the use of fluoroquinolone antimicrobials: an analysis of spontaneous reports and fluoroquinolone consumption data from three italian regions. Drug Saf 2003;26:109. [PMID: 12534327]

Rees JD, et al.: Current concepts in the management of tendon disorders. Rheumatology (Oxford) 2006;45:508. [PMID: 16490749]

Heel Pain, Plantar

ICD-9: 729.5

- **Essentials of Diagnosis**
  - Very common complaint, associated with physical activity; most common cause is plantar fasciitis; may be acute but is more often chronic
  - Pain occurs in the morning with first steps, or after resting
  - Tenderness at the plantar medial aspect of the heel is usually quite localized
  - Radiographs may show a spur at the origin of the fascia, but it is not an acute finding

- **Differential Diagnosis**
  - Atrophy of the heel pad
  - Post-traumatic injury (ie, calcaneal fracture)
  - Lumbar radiculopathy
  - Tarsal tunnel syndrome
  - Entrapment of the nerve of Baxter (nerve to abductor digiti quinti)
  - Sever disease (calcaneal apophysitis) in younger patients

- **Treatment**
  - Plantar fasciitis is treated with NSAIDs, stretching exercises, resilient soft-heeled shoes, and night splinting to keep the Achilles tendon and plantar fascia stretched out overnight; casting and steroid injection can help in refractory cases
  - Surgery to release the medial fascia is ~75% effective; complete rupture of the plantar fascia is a severe, debilitating complication of partial plantar fascia release; extracorporeal shock wave therapy has demonstrated some efficacy
  - Nerve entrapment (ie, tarsal tunnel or entrapment of Baxter nerve) can be surgically released with good results

- **Pearl**

Advise patients that plantar fasciitis can take months to resolve and surgery is not indicated for a minimum of 9 mo.

References

Digiovanni BF, et al.: Plantar fascia-specific stretching exercise improves outcomes in patients with chronic plantar fasciitis. A prospective clinical trial with two-year follow-up. J Bone Joint Surg Am 2006;88:1775. [PMID: 16882901]

Roos E, et al.: Foot orthoses for the treatment of plantar fasciitis. Foot Ankle Int 2006;27:606. [PMID: 16919213]

Sems A, et al.: Extracorporeal shock wave therapy in the treatment of chronic tendinopathies. J Am Acad Orthop Surg 2006;14:195. [PMID: 16585361]

Keratotic Disorders of the Plantar Skin (Callosities)

ICD-9: 700

- **Essentials of Diagnosis**
  - Callosities result from friction and pressure over bony prominences
  - Frequently occur on the plantar surface below the second or third metatarsal head, due to excessively long metatarsals or to splaying of the foot with loss of the transverse arch of the forefoot
  - Assess posture of the foot, presence of deformities, joint mobility, neurovascular status, and degree of callus formation
  - Large intractable calluses can become quite symptomatic and, especially in diabetic patients, may ulcerate
  - Weight-bearing radiographs may show the offending bony prominence

- **Differential Diagnosis**
  - Plantar wart
  - Aging of the foot with loss of transverse arch
  - Rheumatoid arthritis
  - Hypermobile first ray
  - Post-traumatic stiffness
  - Osteoarthritis of the interphalangeal joints

- **Treatment**
  - Cause of the callus dictates treatment
  - Use a wide, soft, lace-up shoe with metatarsal support for mild and early cases; shaving the callus helps temporarily relieve the pain
  - Surgery to remove the associated bony prominence or to correct deformities in intractable or severe cases; metatarsal osteotomies or condylectomies may remove plantar callosities

- **Pearl**

A radiograph with a metal marker over the callus will pinpoint the bony prominence.

References

Feibel JB, et al.: Lesser metatarsal osteotomies. A biomechanical approach to metatarsalgia. Foot Ankle Clin 2001;6:473. [PMID: 11692493]

Mann RA, Mann JA: Keratotic disorders of the plantar skin. Instr Course Lect 2004;53:287. [PMID: 15116622]

8

Hand Problems

Paronychia

ICD-9: 681.02

- ■ Essentials of Diagnosis

  - Paronychia is inflammation of the nail fold (the gutter along the radial and ulnar borders of the nail)
  - It is the most common digital infection and often occurs in people whose hands are immersed in water for long periods
  - It also may be associated with nail cosmetics
  - Infections can be acute or chronic
  - Acute infection is usually with *Staphylococcus aureus*; begins as a cellulitis and progresses to an abscess at the nail margin
  - Chronic infections most often involve *Candida* species

- ■ Differential Diagnosis

  - Felon
  - Mucous cyst
  - Subungual exostosis
  - Herpetic whitlow
  - Longitudinal melanonychia

- ■ Treatment

  - Treatment for acute infection begins with warm soaks and oral antibiotics
  - Incision and drainage is required after an abscess forms
  - Partial nail removal may be necessary to decompress the abscess
  - Treatment of chronic infection includes antimicrobial agents and maintenance of dry hands, and may require nail removal

- ■ Pearl

Chronic infection is often associated with biting of nails and emotional stress.

References

Dahdah MJ, Scher RK: Nail diseases related to nail cosmetics. Dermatol Clin 2006;24:233. [PMID: 16677969]
Yates YJ, Concannon MJ: Fungal infections of the perionychium. Hand Clin 2002;18:631, vi; discussion 643. [PMID: 12516978]

Bennett Fracture

ICD-9: 815.01

- ■ Essentials of Diagnosis
  - Intra-articular fracture of the base of the first metacarpal in which the small volar fragment remains attached to the trapezium and the thumb and first metacarpal are displaced proximally and radially
  - Metacarpal shaft is displaced by forces of the extrinsic thumb extensors and abductor pollicis longus muscles

- ■ Differential Diagnosis
  - Intra-articular Y or T fracture (Rolando)
  - Extra-articular fracture (transverse or oblique)
  - Epiphyseal fracture
  - Thumb dislocations

- ■ Treatment
  - Acute fractures often are reduced by traction and pressure on the proximal metacarpal, with slight pronation; 30 degrees angulation, up to 2 mm intra-articular displacement is acceptable
  - Because displacement of the fracture is caused by the pull of the abductor pollicis longus, the fracture typically requires reduction and fixation
  - The reduction may then be stabilized by percutaneous pin fixation through the metacarpal shaft into either the lip fragment or the trapezium
  - Apply a spica cast for 4–6 weeks
  - Perform open reduction and internal fixation if adequate reduction cannot be obtained, if there is >2 mm displacement, or if a small fragment comprises >25% of the articular surface

- ■ Pearl

Adequate or near anatomic reduction is essential to maintain function.

References

Lutz M, et al.: Closed reduction transarticular Kirschner wire fixation versus open reduction internal fixation in the treatment of Bennett's fracture dislocation. J Hand Surg [Br] 2003;28:142. [PMID: 12631486]

Sawaizumi T, et al.: Percutaneous leverage pinning in the treatment of Bennett's fracture. J Orthop Sci 2005;10:27. [PMID: 15666119]

Bite Injuries

ICD-9: 906.5 Animal; 906.3 Cat; 906.0 Dog; 928.3 Human (accidental); 968.7 Human (assault); 989.5 Spiders, etc

- ■ Essentials of Diagnosis
  - Initially may appear harmless but can inoculate deep tissues with virulent organisms
  - Dog bite: consider *Pasteurella multocida*, *Staphylococcus aureus*, viridans streptococci, *Capnocytophaga canimorsus*, and oral anaerobes
  - Cat bite: infection develops within 24 h; often harbors *P multocida* and other species found in dogs
  - Human bite: often from fist striking tooth; penetrates skin, subcutaneous tissue, extensor tendon, and capsule of metacarpophalangeal (MCP) joint; consider *Eikenella corrodens*, viridans streptococci, group A streptococci, *S aureus*, *Bacteroides*, *Fusobacterium*, *Actinomycetes*, spirochetes
  - Brown recluse spider bite: causes full-thickness skin loss and rapidly spreading erythema with surrounding pallor and cyanosis

- ■ Differential Diagnosis
  - Brown recluse bite: pyoderma gangrenosum
  - MCP septic arthritis

- ■ Treatment
  - Cat or dog bite: incision and drainage; penicillin V, ceftriaxone, tetracycline
  - Human bite: incision and drainage ± arthrotomy if MCP involvement is suspected; begin broad-spectrum IV antibiotics followed by oral penicillin, ampicillin, amoxicillin-clavulanate, and tetanus prophylaxis as indicated
  - Brown recluse bite: early, wide local excision; treatment with dapsone and antibiotics may reduce prevalence of secondary infections and need for surgery
  - Consider rabies vaccine and immune globulin for bites from animals at high risk for rabies (ie, bats, coyotes, raccoons)

- ■ Pearl

Bites distal to the wrist are at higher risk for malignant infections due to the proximity of superficial spaces, flexor tendons, and joints; be wary of the benign wound over the MCP.

References

Rittner AV, et al.: Best evidence topic report. Are antibiotics indicated following human bites? Emerg Med J 2005;22:654. [PMID: 16113192]

Stefanopoulos PK, Tarantzopoulou AD: Facial bite wounds: management update. Int J Oral Maxillofac Surg 2005;34:464. [PMID: 16053863]

Boutonniere Deformity

ICD-9: 736.21

- ■ Essentials of Diagnosis
  - • Proximal interphalangeal (PIP) joint flexion and distal interphalangeal (DIP) hyperextension secondary to central slip disruption on the middle phalanx (laceration, closed rupture, synovitis of PIP joint)
  - • Initial injury may go unrecognized because the finger may function near normally for a few weeks until the PIP joint "buttonholes" through the lateral bands of the extensor mechanism; this basically locks the PIP joint in flexion, resulting in contracture

- ■ Differential Diagnosis
  - • Rheumatoid arthritis
  - • Phalangeal fracture, dislocation
  - • Sagittal band disruption

- ■ Treatment
  - • Treat an acutely lacerated central slip with direct repair and pinning of the joint in full extension for 3–6 wk
  - • Treat acute, closed ruptures of the central slip by splinting the PIP joint in full extension for 6 wk
  - • Delayed treatment: prolonged splinting with Capener splint, or Joint Jack splint versus serial casting; patients with delayed diagnosis may develop fixed flexion contracture of PIP joint

- ■ Pearl

Subluxated lateral bands and unopposed flexor digitorum profundus are the main deforming forces.

References

Peterson JJ, Bancroft LW: Injuries of the fingers and thumb in the athlete. Clin Sports Med 2006;25:527. [PMID: 16798141]

Towfigh H, Gruber P: Surgical treatment of the boutonniere deformity. Oper Orthop Traumatol 2005;17:66. [PMID: 16007379]

Epidermoid Inclusion Cyst

ICD-9: 706.2

■ Essentials of Diagnosis

- Results from proliferation of epidermal cells within a circumscribed space of the dermis
- Appears as a firm, round, mobile, flesh-colored to yellow or white subcutaneous nodule of variable size; a central pore or punctum is an inconsistent finding that may tether the cyst to the overlying epidermis and from which a thick cheesy material can sometimes be expressed
- Manifests in various ways on the extremities; when cysts occur subungually, they can cause changes in the nails (eg, onycholysis, subungual hyperkeratosis) that may be mistaken for psoriasis or onychomycosis; cysts on the distal portions of the digits may extend into the terminal phalanx
- Radiographs of cysts on the distal phalanges may show well-defined osteolytic lesions outlined by a fine rim of bone

■ Differential Diagnosis

- Calcinosis cutis
- Dermoid cyst
- Gardner syndrome
- Lipoma
- Milia

■ Treatment

- Asymptomatic epidermoid cysts do not need to be treated
- Uninfected, inflamed cysts may respond to an intralesional injection of triamcinolone
- For cysts considered to be infected, incision and drainage followed by treatment with antistaphylococcal oral antibiotics is recommended

■ Pearl

The major pitfall in managing epidermoid cysts is failure to diagnose an associated malignancy. Therefore, removal is recommended for any cyst behaving in an unusual way (eg, rapid growth). In turn, all excised cysts should be sent for pathologic analysis.

Reference

Lee HE, et al.: Comparison of the surgical outcomes of punch incision and elliptical excision in treating epidermal inclusion cysts: a prospective, randomized study. Dermatol Surg 2006;32:520. [PMID: 16681659]

Felon

ICD-9: 681.01

- **Essentials of Diagnosis**
  - Felons are closed-space infections of the fingertip pulp
  - Wooden splinters or minor cuts are common predisposing causes, yet no history of injury exists in over half of patients; infection also may spread from a paronychia
  - Initial minor injury causes cellulitis, which is first confined by tough fibrous septa that break up pulp into tiny compartments
  - Felons are characterized by throbbing pain, tension, and edema of the fingertip pulp

- **Differential Diagnosis**
  - Cellulitis
  - Herpetic whitlow
  - Paronychia

- **Treatment**
  - Adequate early treatment can prevent an abscess
  - Decompress to preserve venous flow whenever tension is present, whether or not a frank abscess has formed
  - Perform a midline longitudinal incision of the pad if the infection is pointing there, because this is least likely to injure nerves or circulation; for diffuse lesions, use an incision on the ulnar side of the finger (except for the thumb and little) and be sure to divide septa that may be preventing egress of the purulent material
  - Administer antibiotics with activity against staphylococcal and streptococcal organisms
  - Splint and elevate finger

- **Pearl**

Herpetic whitlow can closely mimic a felon and will not respond to incision and drainage—suspect this condition in medical or dental personnel.

References

Canales FL, et al.: The treatment of felons and paronychias. Hand Clinics 1989;5:515. [PMID: 2681234]

Clark DC: Common acute hand infections. Am Fam Physician 2003;68:2167. [PMID: 14677662]

Connolly B, et al.: Methicillin-resistant Staphylococcus aureus in a finger felon. J Hand Surg [Am] 2000;25:173. [PMID: 10642489]

Ganglion Cyst

ICD-9: 727.41

- Essentials of Diagnosis
  - Comprises 50–70% of all hand masses
  - Most commonly found on wrist, digital flexor sheath, interphalangeal (IP) joint, ankle, foot, and knee
  - Probably caused by a hole in an adjacent joint capsule or synovial sheath
  - Filled with a gelatinous mucoid material
  - Nonpainful when large, sometimes painful when small; may be transilluminated
  - If patient has pain, determine whether it is coming from the cyst; often the cyst is the obvious abnormality, and pain is originating from some other cause (eg, ligament injuries of the wrist, osteoarthritis, etc)

- Differential Diagnosis
  - Giant cell tumor of tendon sheath
  - Pigmented villonodular synovitis
  - Lipoma
  - Synovial sarcoma
  - Cavernous hemangioma

- Treatment
  - Aspiration and steroid injection alleviates ~80% of ganglion cysts, but there is a high recurrence rate
  - Symptomatic cysts that do not respond to steroid injection can be excised, taking the entire stalk

- Pearl

The most common location is the radial and dorsal aspect of the wrist, where excision can remove the dorsal portion of the scapholunate ligament and cause iatrogenic scapholunate dissociation.

Reference

Nahra ME, Bucchieri JS: Ganglion cysts and other tumor related conditions of the hand and wrist. Hand Clin 2004;20:249. [PMID: 15275684]

Fingertip Injuries

ICD-9: 927.3 Crush; 834.02 Dislocation; 886.1 Amputation; 883.0 Laceration

- **Essentials of Diagnosis**
  - Key history: mechanism of injury, occupation and hobbies, length of time since injury; tetanus immunization status
  - Various types: crush versus sharp injuries, nail or nail bed, and bone involvement; amputation or partial amputation; viability of tip
  - Assess for presence of foreign body (ie, lawn mower injury)
  - Radiographs may be necessary either to assess alignment of distal phalanx fractures or to detect presence of foreign bodies

- **Differential Diagnosis**
  - Nail bed injury
  - Amputation

- **Treatment**
  - Lacerations: clean wound and inspect (typically done under digital block and tourniquet); suture simple lacerations
  - Remove nail and inspect matrix when fingertip injuries disrupt it; repair nail matrix with small absorbable suture (eg, 6-0 chromic)
  - Subungual hematoma: decompress acute, painful hematomas with an 18-gauge needle
  - Fingertip amputations: goal is minimal tenderness, adequate sensation, satisfactory appearance; length is important but not at the expense of function; most can be handled acutely by debridement, removal of exposed bone, and dressing
  - Various methods are used for amputation injuries, including simple revision amputation, full- or partial-thickness skin grafts, local flaps, distal flaps, and neurovascular island pedicle flaps

- **Pearl**

Untreated nail bed lacerations may lead to subsequent nail deformities.

References

Chang J, et al.: Fingertip injuries. Clin Occup Environ Med 2006;5:413. [PMID: 16647658]

Datiashvili RO, et al.: Solutions to challenging digital replantations. Clin Plast Surg 2007;34:167. [PMID: 17418668]

Evans D, Bernadis C: A new classification for fingertip injuries. J Hand Surg [Br] 2000;25:58. [PMID: 9043584]

Lee LP, et al.: A simple and efficient treatment for fingertip injuries. J Hand Surg [Br] 1995;20:63. [PMID: 10763726]

Ulnar Neuropathy

ICD-9: 354.2

■ Essentials of Diagnosis

- Multiple sites of entrapment; most common is the cubital tunnel (and others near the elbow), then canal of Guyon (at the wrist)
- Decreased sensation in ulnar nerve distribution; Tinel sign is present at area of entrapment; in severe cases, muscle atrophy
- Weakness in ulnar-innervated intrinsic muscles of the hand (Froment sign); more proximal lesions cause weakness of the flexor digitorum longus to the ring and little finger
- EMG/NCS can help with diagnosis and localization

■ Differential Diagnosis

- Ulnar nerve entrapment near the elbow
- Ulnar nerve entrapment at canal of Guyon
- Cervical radiculopathy
- Ganglion impinging on nerve
- Hook of Hamate fracture
- Synovitis
- Medial epicondylitis (can occur concurrently with cubital tunnel syndrome)

■ Treatment

- Conservative treatment for elbow entrapment requires protecting the nerve from stretch and compression, using either an elbow pad or a splint at 45 degrees of flexion, worn continuously or at night; similarly, if compression is at the wrist, a wrist splint is used
- Medial epicondylectomy, submuscular or subcutaneous transposition, and external neurolysis are surgical approaches for the ulnar nerve at the elbow if conservative measures fail; Guyon canal release and neurolysis are possible treatments for distal entrapments

■ Pearl

Entrapments at the wrist demonstrate sensory decrease only in the ulnar $1\frac{1}{2}$ fingers, because the sensory branches to the hypothenar eminence arise from the ulnar nerve proximal to the wrist.

References

Biggs M, Curtis JA: Randomized, prospective study comparing ulnar neurolysis in situ with submuscular transposition. Neurosurgery 2006;58:296; discussion 296. [PMID: 16462483]

Corwin HM: Compression neuropathies of the upper extremity. Clin Occup Environ Med 2006;5:333. [PMID: 16647652]

Anterior Interosseous Nerve Syndrome

ICD-9: 354.1

- **Essentials of Diagnosis**
  - Anterior interosseous nerve (AIN) is a branch of the medial nerve
  - AIN syndrome is caused by compression of the nerve by the deep head of the pronator teres, origin of the flexor digitorum superficialis, palmaris profundus, flexor carpi radialis, or "Ganzer" muscle (accessory head of the flexor pollicis longus [FDL])
  - Patient complains of inability to flex the thumb interphalangeal joint as well as the index finger distal interphalangeal joint (AIN innervates the radial two flexor digitorum profundus, FPL, and pronator quadratus muscles)
  - Pain and numbness are not usually characteristic of this syndrome (as they might be in pronator syndrome)
  - EMG/NCG can be helpful in confirming the diagnosis
  - MRI can be helpful for defining the location of entrapment

- **Differential Diagnosis**
  - Tendon rupture
  - Parsonage-Turner syndrome (viral brachial neuritis) in bilateral cases
  - Cervical radiculopathy
  - Peripheral neuropathy
  - Compression can rarely be caused by a mass (eg, lipoma or sarcoma)

- **Treatment**
  - Exploration and decompression of compressing structures is required if observation fails to show improvement (usually effective if done within 3–6 mo of the onset of symptoms

- **Pearl**

Patients usually only complain of weakness, unlike pronator syndrome in which pain and numbness are common.

Reference

Kim S et al.: Role of magnetic resonance imaging in entrapment and compressive neuropathy—what, where and how to see the peripheral nerves on the musculoskeletal magnetic resonance image: part 2. Upper extremity. Eur Radiol 2006;17:509. [PMID: 16572333]

Posterior Interosseous Nerve Syndrome

ICD-9: 354.3

- Essentials of Diagnosis
  - Posterior interosseous nerve (PIN) is a branch of the radial nerve
  - PIN syndrome is caused by compression of the nerve by the superficial head of the supinator at the arcade of Frohse, or in the supinator
  - Patient has tenderness over the PIN, usually 3–6 cm distal to the lateral epicondyle (vs lateral epicondylitis)
  - Patient cannot extend all digits and has weakness in wrist extension due to possible involvement of extensor carpi ulnaris
  - Numbness is not a characteristic of this syndrome; it is a pure motor nerve syndrome
  - EMG/NCG can be helpful in confirming diagnosis

- Differential Diagnosis
  - Lateral epicondylitis
  - Tendon rupture
  - Iatrogenic, from treatment of proximal radius fracture
  - Ganglia, lipomas
  - Cervical radiculopathy
  - Peripheral neuropathy

- Treatment
  - Exploration and decompression of compressing structures is required if observation fails to show improvement

- Pearl

MRI may be helpful in delineating masses in the nerve area at the elbow.

References

Arle JE, Zager EL: Surgical treatment of common entrapment neuropathies in the upper limbs. Muscle Nerve 2000;23:1160. [PMID: 10918251]

Henry, M, Stutz C: A unified approach to radial tunnel syndrome and lateral tendinosis. Tech Hand Up Extrem Surg 2006;10:200. [PMID: 17159475]

Carpal Tunnel Syndrome

ICD-9: 354.0

- **Essentials of Diagnosis**
  - Compression of median nerve in the carpal tunnel (space on palmar aspect of wrist bounded by scaphoid, trapezium, capitate, hook of hamate, pisiform, and transverse carpal ligament)
  - Often idiopathic but associated with pregnancy, hypothyroidism, diabetes, amyloidosis, overuse phenomena, trauma, and tumors in the carpal tunnel
  - Numbness in the median nerve distribution; pain awakens patient from sleep; wrist-flexed activities are uncomfortable and elicit symptoms
  - Tinel sign, Phalen wrist flexion test (negative after 1 min), weak opposition, or thenar atrophy may be present
  - Most sensitive test is carpal compression (direct compression over carpal tunnel for 60 s); sensory exam is very helpful
  - Obtain radiographs, including a carpal tunnel view, to rule out bony causes of carpal tunnel syndrome (CTS)
  - EMG/NCS can help differentiate CTS from other entities but findings are often normal in early CTS
  - Atrophy of thenar muscles is a sign of advanced disease

- **Differential Diagnosis**
  - Cervical radiculopathy
  - Peripheral neuropathy
  - Proximal median nerve compression syndromes: pronator syndrome, anterior interosseus syndrome

- **Treatment**
  - Begins with splinting in slight extension and evaluation of causes other than idiopathic; steroid injections in the carpal tunnel can help reduce symptoms for a period of time
  - Surgical treatment is indicated when conservative therapy is unsuccessful; the transverse carpal ligament can be divided by open surgery or by endoscopic surgery; success rates are high

- **Pearl**

Check sensation on the two sides of the pulp of the ring finger. The ulnar nerve innervates the ulnar side and the median nerve, the radial side. Patients can often discern a difference.

References

van den Bekerom MP, et al.: Outcome of open versus endoscopic approach for the surgical treatment of carpal tunnel syndrome. Acta Orthop Belg 2006;72:288. [PMID: 16889140]

Wilder-Smith EP, et al.: Diagnosing carpal tunnel syndrome—clinical criteria and ancillary tests. Nat Clin Pract Neurol 2006;2:366. [PMID: 16932587]

Thoracic Outlet Syndrome

ICD-9: 724.4

- **Essentials of Diagnosis**
  - Bony borders are medial clavicle, first rib, and cervical rib
  - Outlet is formed by anterior scalene (anterior), middle scalene (posterior), and first rib (inferior)
  - Causes: clavicular fracture and hypertrophy; microtrauma causing intrascalene fibrosis; subclavian thrombosis (edema, cyanosis)
  - Compression of brachial plexus, subclavian artery or vein
  - More common in women, with onset of symptoms usually between 20 and 50 y
  - C8–T1 roots are usually affected; pain and paresthesia radiate to medial arm, ulnar distribution symptoms are vague and exacerbated by overhead, abducted position
  - Adson test: turning head to the affected side obliterates radial pulse
  - Wright test: holding shoulder in abduction and external rotation with elbow flexed for 3 min while rapidly opening and closing hand obliterates radial pulse
  - Chest radiographs, shoulder films, EMG/NCS, Doppler studies

- **Differential Diagnosis**
  - C8, T1 cervical radiculopathy
  - Carpal tunnel syndrome, ulnar neuropathy
  - Peripheral neuropathy
  - Connective tissue diseases or infection
  - Rotator cuff instability
  - Brachial neuritis
  - Pancoast tumors
  - Angina
  - Regional pain syndrome

- **Treatment**
  - 75% of patients improve with conservative measures: shoulder girdle strengthening (upper and lower trapezius, erector spinae, serratus anterior), correction of poor posture
  - First rib resection with or without scalenotomy via anterior supraclavicular exposure or the transaxillary approach

- **Pearl**

Cervical ribs are found in 1% of population.

Reference

Huang JH, Zager EL: Thoracic outlet syndrome. Neurosurgery 2004;55:897; discussion 902. [PMID: 15458598]

Flexor Suppurative Tenosynovitis

ICD-9: 727.05 Tenosynovitis of hand; 041 Bacterial infections

- **Essentials of Diagnosis**
  - Patients with infectious flexor tenosynovitis (FT) may present at anytime following a puncture wound or laceration, especially at the finger creases where padding is limited; patients do not always recall having a puncture wound
  - Complaints of pain, redness, fever; pain with motion
  - Physical exam reveals Kanaval signs of flexor tendon sheath infection (finger held in slight flexion, fusiform swelling, tenderness along flexor tendon sheath, pain with passive extension of digit)
  - Lab values may show elevated WBC count and ESR
  - Obtain standard AP and lateral radiographs to rule out bony involvement or foreign body

- **Differential Diagnosis**
  - Inflammatory (nonsuppurative) FT
  - Herpetic whitlow
  - Pyarthrosis
  - Gout
  - Dactylitis
  - Phalanx fracture

- **Treatment**
  - If a patient presents very early (within first 24 h) with suspected infectious FT, medical treatment may initially include IV antibiotics (empiric for streptococci and staphylococci)
  - If unsure of diagnosis, fluid can be aspirated from the tendon sheath, inspected, and sent for Gram stain, cell count, and culture
  - Splinting in interphalangeal extension and metacarpophalangeal flexion; elevation initially until infection is controlled
  - Indications for surgical drainage include history and physical exam findings consistent with acute or chronic FT; early surgical intervention is warranted for immunocompromised or diabetic patients; if medical treatment alone is attempted, inpatient observation for at least 48 h is indicated; surgical drainage is necessary if no obvious improvement has occurred within 12–24 h

- **Pearl**

Pain with any passive extension of the finger(s) is highly suspicious for FT.

Reference

Small LN, Ross JJ: Suppurative tenosynovitis and septic bursitis. Infect Dis Clin North Am 2005;19:991. [PMID: 16297744]

Flexor Tenosynovitis: Trigger Finger & Thumb

ICD-9: 727.03

■ Essentials of Diagnosis

- Congenital form: child with flexed thumb since infancy
- Adult form: flexor tendons to the fingers and thumb develop nodules secondary to trauma
- Pain at site of locking (proximal edge of the A1 [metacarpophalangeal joint level] pulley)
- Palpable nodule in tendon
- Feeling of locking or clicking with flexion-extension
- Patient often feels clicking and pain more distally in the finger than at the level of the A1 pulley

■ Differential Diagnosis

- Dupuytren disease
- Tendon rupture
- Rheumatoid arthritis
- Degenerative joint disease of the finger joints

■ Treatment

- Steroid injection into the sheath is often very helpful
- Surgical release of the pulley is a simple operation that is especially indicated for diabetic patients, in whom conservative treatment is less effective
- Success rate for percutaneous release with steroid injection is twice as effective as steroid injection alone in thumbs

■ Pearl

Steroid injection has a 64% cure rate in patients with primary trigger finger.

References

Maneerit J, et al.: Trigger thumb: results of a prospective randomised study of percutaneous release with steroid injection versus steroid injection alone. J Hand Surg [Br] 2003;28:586. [PMID: 14599834]

Ryzewicz M, Wolf JM: Trigger digits: principles, management, and complications. J Hand Surg [Am] 2006;31:135. [PMID: 16443118]

De Quervain Flexor Tenosynovitis

ICD-9: 727.0

- ■ Essentials of Diagnosis
  - Tenosynovitis may occur in any of the extensor or flexor tendons, throughout their length; De Quervain tenosynovitis occurs at the radial styloid and involves the abductor pollicis longus and extensor pollicis brevis
  - Inflammation is under the retinaculum of the first extensor compartment
  - Patient has a history of pain at the radial side of the wrist with activities in which the thumb is abducted or the wrist is ulnarly deviated
  - Palpation elicits pain at the site of the retinaculum at the radial styloid)
  - Finkelstein test: thumb is put in the palm and enclosed by the fingers; the wrist is abruptly deviated ulnarly; positive test results in pain at the radial side of the wrist

- ■ Differential Diagnosis
  - De Quervain disease of pregnancy
  - Scaphoid fracture
  - Tendon rupture
  - Rheumatoid arthritis

- ■ Treatment
  - Splinting does not cure the problem but provides symptomatic relief
  - Steroid injection into the first extensor compartment is successful in most patients, but as many as 25% need a second injection to get relief, probably because the 2 tendons have separate compartments and the abductor has variable numbers of accessory tendon slips
  - Surgical release of the retinaculum is indicated for patients who do not respond to conservative therapy

- ■ Pearl

De Quervain tenosynovitis may be accompanied by a symptomatic ganglion, or triggering of the tendons in the compartment, or both.

References

Avci S, et al.: Comparison of nonsurgical treatment measures for de Quervain's disease of pregnancy and lactation. J Hand Surg [Am] 2002;27:322. [PMID: 11901392]

Sarikcioglu L, Yildirim FB: Bilateral abductor pollicis longus muscle variation. Case report and review of the literature. Morphologie 2004;88:160. [PMID: 15641655]

High-Pressure Injection Injury

ICD-9: 989.9

- **Essentials of Diagnosis**
  - High pressures involved with injection tools are sufficient to penetrate skin from a distance; contact of the device with the hand is not a prerequisite for injury to occur
  - Typical injury is to an index finger used to clean off the tip of the injection gun; injected material follows the flexor tendons into the palm
  - Grease gun injuries tend to cause fibrosis of soft tissue
  - Paint and paint thinner injuries are severe and tend to cause necrosis of soft tissue with a high associated amputation rate
  - Early on, patient has minimal symptoms with either an innocuous entrance wound or no visible entrance wound
  - Later symptoms include a painful, swollen, and pale digit because of vascular compromise and tissue necrosis

- **Differential Diagnosis**
  - Illicit drug injection
  - Compartment syndrome
  - Ischemic disease

- **Treatment**
  - IV broad-spectrum antibiotics, with splinting, elevation, and analgesia
  - Thorough decompression and debridement are needed urgently to clean injected material from tissues
  - Patient often requires multiple irrigation and debridements
  - Some clinicians advocate leaving the wounds open and letting them close by secondary intention

- **Pearl**

The type, amount, and velocity of injected material are important factors as well as the anatomic location in regard to outcome. The single most important factor is the type of material injected.

Reference

Gonzalez R, Kasdan ML: High pressure injection injuries of the hand. Clin Occup Environ Med 2006;5:407. [PMID: 16647657]

Tendon Laceration: Hand & Wrist

ICD-9: 883.2 Finger; 882.2 Hand

■ Essentials of Diagnosis

- Lacerations of hand or wrist tendons usually involve extensor or flexor tendons; flexor tendon lacerations are more common
- Produces loss of extension or flexion; characteristic posture of fingers can point to lacerated tendons
- Exam should test every tendon and nerve that may be affected; test sensory function before use of local anesthetic
- Radiographs are indicated to rule out foreign body or fracture

■ Differential Diagnosis

- Hand or wrist fracture
- Proximal nerve palsy causing loss of distal function
- Tendon rupture

■ Treatment

- Extensor tendons can often be repaired in the emergency department unless multiple or at the level of the wrist; late repair is also possible; immobilization should be in wrist extension with the metacarpophalangeal (MCP) joints flexed
- Flexor tendon lacerations are more difficult to manage; treatment depends on location of the laceration; both superficial and deep finger flexors may be lacerated; nerve (digital, ulnar, median), artery (radial, ulnar, or both), and wrist flexors may be involved; these cases require operative repair under tourniquet control for optimal results
- Location of flexor tendon laceration is important; zone 1 of flexor surface is distal to insertion of sublimis tendon (middle of middle phalanx); zone 2 is from zone 1 to level of metacarpal head (distal palmar crease); zone 3 is from zone 2 to carpal ligament; zone 4 is carpal canal; zone 5 is proximal to zone 4
- Zone 2 injuries are the most difficult (known as "no man's land" because of historically poor results); improved technique has resulted in better results

■ Pearl

Early motion is the key to obtaining good functional results in flexor tendons. This is less important for extensor tendons.

References

Hung LK, et al.: Active mobilization after flexor tendon repair: comparison of results following injuries in zone 2 and other zones. J Orthop Surg (Hong Kong) 2005;13:158. [PMID: 2324453]

Mowlavi A, et al.: Dynamic versus static splinting of simple zone V and zone VI extensor tendon repairs: a prospective, randomized, controlled study. Plast Reconstr Surg 2005;115:482. [PMID: 15692354]

Intrinsic Muscle Tightness

ICD-9: 719:54

■ Essentials of Diagnosis

- Intrinsic muscles have their origins and insertions within the hand; they include the muscles of the thenar and hypothenar eminences, adductor pollicis, interossei, and lumbricals
- Interosseous and lumbrical muscles flex the metacarpophalangeal (MCP) joints and extend the interphalangeal joints of the fingers
- When contractures are mild, the MCP joints can be passively extended completely, but while they are held extended, the proximal interphalangeal joints cannot be flexed (positive intrinsic tightness test)
- Complete contractures of the intrinsic muscles lead to the "intrinsic-plus" hand

■ Differential Diagnosis

- Fibrosis, post-trauma or infection
- Rheumatoid arthritis
- Postpolio syndrome
- Postcompartment syndrome of the hand
- Closed head injury
- Late nerve injury

■ Treatment

- Releases to lengthen the intrinsics are either at the muscle level or at the lateral bands; the intrinsic tightness test is used intraoperatively to determine the adequacy of the releases

■ Pearl

To test for intrinsic tightness in the rheumatoid hand, the examiner must be sure the MCP joints are reduced. If dislocated, the intrinsics will appear falsely lax.

Reference

Lee FS, Gellman H: Reconstruction of intrinsic hand deformities. Hand Clin 1998;14:499. [PMID: 9742428]

Compartment Syndrome: Hand

ICD-9: 733.7 Sudeck atrophy; 728.89 Muscle ischemia

- **Essentials of Diagnosis**
  - Intrinsic muscles of the hand can be damaged by pressure, causing a Finochietto ischemic contracture
  - Compartment syndrome results from increased pressure in an enclosed anatomic space that inhibits necessary capillary perfusion for intrinsic muscle viability
  - Frequently overlooked because symptoms of pain and swelling also occur with trauma
  - Elevated compartment pressures are caused by swelling and hemorrhage from metacarpal fractures, crush injuries, reperfusion injury, and arteriovenous fistulas as well as a constricting cast, garment, or iatrogenically from excessive tension with a surgical fascial closure
  - Clinical signs ("5 P's"): excessive Pain with palpation or especially *passive muscle motion*, Paresthesias, Pallor, and, in late stages, Pulselessness and Paralysis
  - In obtunded patients, it is mandatory to test compartment pressures with a manometer if compartments appear tense or full; insert measurement device into the midsubstance of the compressed muscle or soft tissue

- **Differential Diagnosis**
  - Crush injury
  - Metacarpal fracture(s)
  - Roller or shear injury

- **Treatment**
  - Remove casts and circumferential dressings; measure compartment pressures; splint or immobilize fractures
  - Perform fasciotomies (surgical release of constricting fascial planes) to decompress soft tissues in patients with compartment pressures >40 mm Hg from diastolic blood pressure and in all obtunded patients or if compartment syndrome is suspected, irrespective of results of pressure measurements
  - Delayed treatment results in "intrinsic-plus" deformity

- **Pearl**

IV fluids and especially imaging contrast material can cause compartment syndrome when extravasation occurs.

References

Ortiz JA, Jr., Berger RA: Compartment syndrome of the hand and wrist. Hand Clin 1998;14:405. [PMID: 9742420]

Ouellette EA: Compartment syndromes in obtunded patients. Hand Clin 1998;14:431. [PMID: 9742422]

Volkmann Ischemic Contracture

ICD-9: 958.6

- **Essentials of Diagnosis**
  - Caused by the late residua of an acute compartment syndrome in the forearm
  - Ischemic death of muscle tissue results in fibrosis and sometimes neural damage; fibrous tissue contracts with time, causing shortening of the associated tendons
  - Damage can range from mild, producing minimal muscle tightness on physical exam, to complete death of the muscle with no function of the involved muscles
  - If the volar side of the forearm is involved, finger flexors are tight and do not straighten passively; if both volar and dorsal sides are involved, clawing is a result
  - Elbow flexion, forearm pronation, wrist flexion, thumb flexion, finger metacarpophalangeal extension, and interphalangeal flexion are often present

- **Differential Diagnosis**
  - Neural injury to the median or ulnar nerve

- **Treatment**
  - Prevention, by alleviating acute compartment syndrome before muscle death occurs, is the best treatment
  - In patients with some function, stretching with occupational therapy, and tendon lengthening to put the active motion in the most functional position, can be performed
  - Neurolysis of major nerves and tendon transfers are other treatment options

- **Pearl**

Compartment syndrome release after death of the muscle exposes the dead muscle to the risk of infection.

References

Botte MJ, et al.: Volkmann's ischemic contracture of the upper extremity. Hand Clin 1998;14:483. [PMID: 9742427]

Stevanovich M, Sharpe F: Management of established Volkmann's contracture of the forearm in children. Hand Clin 2006;22:99. [PMID: 16504782]

Kienböck Disease

ICD-9: 733.49

- ■ Essentials of Diagnosis
  - • Results from ischemic necrosis of the lunate in the wrist
  - • More common in patients with abnormally short ulnas (at wrist); most often seen in patients between 15 and 40 y of age; usually unilateral
  - • Patient presents with wrist pain that radiates to the forearm, wrist stiffness, swelling or tenderness over the lunate, and decreased grip strength
  - • Radiographs show sclerosis of the lunate and progressive loss of height with worsening disease
  - • In early stages, MRI shows decreased vascularity

- ■ Differential Diagnosis
  - • Carpal bone fracture
  - • Carpal instability
  - • Distal radioulnar joint pain (ulnocarpal impaction syndrome)
  - • Triangular fibrocartilage complex tear

- ■ Treatment
  - • Splinting can provide symptomatic relief but is not effective in changing the course of the disease
  - • Surgical shortening of the radius, proximal row carpectomy, or carpal fusion can be performed, depending on severity of disease
  - • Vascularized bone graft techniques have been used with some success but are technically demanding

- ■ Pearl

Arthroscopy can be used to evaluate the extent of damage to the lunate and associated articular surfaces.

Reference

Bain GI, Begg M: Arthroscopic assessment and classification of Kienbock's disease. Tech Hand Up Extrem Surg 2006;10:8. [PMID: 16628114]

Profundus (Flexor Digitorum Longus) Avulsion

ICD-9: 842.13

- **Essentials of Diagnosis**
  - Flexor tendon injuries distal to the insertion of the flexor digitorum superficialis are often closed injuries (and can be missed); lacerations and crush injuries may occur
  - Profundus avulsion occurs in sports as a result of forced extension of a flexed distal interphalangeal (DIP) joint; also called *rugger jersey finger*
  - Most common in the ring finger
  - Exam reveals loss of DIP flexion and sometimes a palpable mass in the palm
  - Distal phalanx may retract into the palm
  - Radiographs are required to determine if a bony fragment was avulsed

- **Differential Diagnosis**
  - Distal phalanx fracture
  - Osteoarthritis deformity

- **Treatment**
  - Avulsions seen within 10 days require operative reattachment of the tendon; after 10 days, treatment is individualized and depends on where the tendon stump is located (ie, palm vs digit), time from injury, and functional demands of the patient
  - Other options include DIP fusion, free grafting, and no treatment

- **Pearl**

Ultrasound can be helpful in the diagnosis of avulsions when no fracture is present.

References

Cohen SB, et al.: Use of ultrasound in determining treatment for avulsion of the flexor digitorum profundus (rugger jersey finger): a case report. Am J Orthop 2004;33:546. [PMID: 15603514]

Tuttle HG, et al.: Tendon avulsion injuries of the distal phalanx. Clin Orthop Relat Res 2006;445:157. [PMID: 16601414]

Swan-Neck Deformity

ICD-9: 736.22

- **Essentials of Diagnosis**
  - Deformity characterized by hyperextension of proximal inter-phalangeal (PIP) joint, flexion of distal interphalangeal (DIP) joint, and metacarpophalangeal (MCP) joint flexion
  - Caused by attenuation or rupture of the extensor tendon insertion into the distal phalanx
  - Functional loss associated with this deformity is related to decreased range of motion at the interphalangeal joints
  - Causes include untreated mallet deformity, volar plate laxity, ligamentous laxity, and malunion of a fracture of the middle phalanx
  - Most common mechanism in rheumatoid arthritis is intrinsic tightness with associated MCP synovitis
  - True swan-neck deformity does not affect the thumb

- **Differential Diagnosis**
  - Mallet finger
  - Osteoarthritis
  - Rheumatoid arthritis
  - Boutonniere deformity

- **Treatment**
  - Treatment depends on the cause of the problem
  - In rheumatoid arthritis, if function is compromised, early conservative management includes finger splinting of the PIP to prevent hyperextension and DIP arthrodesis as the treatment of choice; intrinsic release may be helpful in more severe cases
  - PIP joint arthroplasty can also be performed if tendons are intact, when the joint is arthritic
  - Flexible swan-neck, resulting from traumatic mallet finger can be treated with ligament reconstruction

- **Pearl**

Less common in rheumatoid arthritis than from other causes.

References

Bendre AA, et al.: Mallet finger. J Am Acad Orthop Surg 2005;13:336. [PMID: 16148359]

Tuttle HG, et al.: Tendon avulsion injuries of the distal phalanx. Clin Orthop Relat Res 2006;445:157. [PMID: 16601414]

Mallet Finger

ICD-9: 736.1

- ■ Essentials of Diagnosis
  - Loss of full, active extension of the distal interphalangeal (DIP) joint, resulting in unopposed flexor digitorum longus action to pull the distal phalanx into flexion
  - Loss of extension can be due to avulsion of the tendon with or without a fragment of bone, or rupture or laceration of the tendon inserting on the distal phalanx
  - Traumatic (except for rheumatoid arthritis)
  - Patient often presents late, weeks after the injury
  - Radiographs are necessary to determine if an intra-articular fracture is present

- ■ Differential Diagnosis
  - Distal phalanx fracture
  - Dislocation of the distal joint

- ■ Treatment
  - Injuries are usually closed and can be treated with *continuous* splinting of the DIP joint in full extension for 8 wk
  - Articular fragments if small (ie, <33% of the joint surface) can be ignored and treated as if ligament injuries
  - Single large fracture fragments can be treated operatively to reduce the fracture
  - Joint is usually pinned in extension
  - Chronic mallet finger can often be successfully treated with splinting; if splinting is unsuccessful and the amount of finger flexion is unacceptable, finger fusion is an option

- ■ Pearl

Surgical management is reserved for patients who cannot work with a splint in place or those who have large fragments or dislocated joints.

References

Bendre AA, et al.: Mallet finger. J Am Acad Orthop Surg 2005;13:336. [PMID: 16148359]

Kalainov DM, et al.: Nonsurgical treatment of closed mallet finger fractures. J Hand Surg [Am] 2005;30:580. [PMID: 15925171]

Gamekeeper's Thumb

ICD-9: 842.01

- **Essentials of Diagnosis**
  - Laxity of the ulnar collateral ligament (UCL) of the thumb metacarpophalangeal (MCP) joint
  - Caused by any repetitive abrupt abduction force on the thumb that stretches or ruptures the ligament
  - If undisplaced, the ligament ends stay approximated; if displaced, the adductor aponeurosis isolates the ligament end from the proximal phalanx (Stener lesion)
  - Occasionally, when the UCL ruptures, the adductor hallucis brevis muscle or fascia becomes interposed between the 2 ends of the UCL (Stener lesion); these injuries do not heal with conservative treatment and require surgical repair
  - Physical exam reveals a lack of end point in ligament testing in abduction of the MCP joint
  - Radiographs reveal 15 degrees of abduction angulation *more* than the opposite side in complete rupture; may also reveal an avulsion fracture that has the ligament attached to it
  - MRI may be helpful in defining pathology

- **Differential Diagnosis**
  - Radial collateral injury to the thumb
  - Spontaneously reduced dislocation of the MCP joint
  - Skier's thumb (traumatic rupture of the UCL [nonrepetitive]; although this term is sometimes used synonymously with gamekeeper's thumb, in gamekeeper's thumb rupture occurs as a result of repetitive microtrauma to the UCL)

- **Treatment**
  - Partial tears of the UCL can be treated with a thumb spica; complete acute tears, which are usually displaced from the proximal phalanx, should be repaired surgically
  - Late repairs and reconstructions provide better results than MCP arthrodesis

- **Pearl**

Traumatic injuries to the thumb can injure either the radial (often missed) or ulnar collateral ligament; however, injury to the UCL is much more common. Failure to treat UCL injuries will result in key pinch weakness.

Reference

Fairhurst M, Hansen L: Treatment of "Gamekeeper's thumb" by reconstruction of the ulnar collateral ligament. J Hand Surg [Br] 2002;27:542. [PMID: 12475512]

Dupuytren Disease

ICD-9: 728.6

- **Essentials of Diagnosis**
  - Progressive nodular thickening on the fascia of the palmar surface of the hand; associated with Peyronie disease (penis), Ledderhose disease (plantar foot), alcohol, smoking, and diabetes
  - More common in men, with usual age of onset 40–60 y; predisposition in patients of northern European ancestry and occasionally Asians
  - Causes gradual contracture of the palmar fascia, resulting in metacarpophalangeal (MCP) and proximal interphalangeal (PIP) joint contractures; usually the little finger is worst
  - Symptoms of finger(s) "catching" in pockets, cosmetic complaints, shaking hands, and occasionally, with severe cases of contracture, hygiene of the finger creases

- **Differential Diagnosis**
  - Non-Dupuytren palmar fascial disease
  - Burn scarring and flexion contractures
  - Traumatic scarring and flexion contractures

- **Treatment**
  - Nonoperative treatment is efficacious in milder forms of the disease when joint flexion contractures are small
  - Surgical treatment is indicated to remove the fascia (fasciectomy) causing the contractures; joint contracture of 30 degrees at the MCP or any contracture at the PIP joint is the indication for surgery
  - In severe, neglected cases or cases with neurovascular compromise or extreme stiffness, amputation of the little finger may be necessary
  - Surgery is risky because neurovascular structures are intimately adherent to the nodular fascia in Dupuytren contractures

- **Pearl**

Early surgery prevents severe contractures but is associated with a high rate of recurrence of the disease.

References

Rayan GM, Moore J: Non-Dupuytren's disease of the palmar fascia. J Hand Surg [Br] 2005;30:551. [PMID: 16203068]

Reilly RM, et al.: A retrospective review of the management of Dupuytren's nodules. J Hand Surg [Am] 2005;30:1014. [PMID: 16182060]

Foreign Body in Soft Tissue

ICD-9: 729.6

- Essentials of Diagnosis
  - Foreign bodies in the soft tissue are frequent, especially in the hand and foot
  - Needles, nails, thorns, glass, and stone are commonly embedded
  - Acutely, the laceration or puncture may not reveal the foreign body; chronically, the laceration may drain or heal but be sensitive to palpation
  - Occasionally, a foreign body becomes walled off from the surrounding tissue and forms an inclusion cyst
  - Many foreign bodies can be visualized on radiographs

- Differential Diagnosis
  - Laceration or puncture

- Treatment
  - Unless the foreign body is easily palpable or visible, conditions should be optimized to remove it
  - A tourniquet is best employed for hand or foot exploration to minimize bleeding, optimize visibility, and minimize risk to neurovascular structures; anesthesia helps for the same reasons
  - For foreign bodies that are visible on radiographs, C-arm imaging is very helpful; for other radiolucent materials, ultrasound guidance is helpful
  - If the foreign body cannot be located, it is also acceptable to leave the wound open, treat the patient with antibiotics, and allow the body to localize the foreign body by forming a capsule around it; the foreign body can then be removed electively, with the tissue reaction pointing to the location

- Pearl

Ultrasound is a helpful modality that should be used to guide the acute removal of foreign bodies.

Reference

Graham DD Jr: Ultrasound in the emergency department: detection of wooden foreign bodies in the soft tissues. J Emerg Med 2002;22:75. [PMID: 11809560]

Metacarpal Neck Fracture

ICD-9: 815.04 Neck; 815.01 Base of first metacarpal; 815.03 Shaft

- **Essentials of Diagnosis**
    - The fifth metacarpal is the most common metacarpal neck fracture; also known as a *boxer's fracture*
    - Usually caused by direct impact on the distal end of the metacarpal, causing apex dorsal angulation with comminution of the volar cortex, just proximal to the metacarpophalangeal (MCP) joint
    - History of trauma; pain and swelling at the end of the metacarpal
    - Tenderness and possibly crepitus at the fracture site
    - Pain with motion of the MCP joint
    - Radiographs confirm the diagnosis

- **Differential Diagnosis**
    - Metacarpal head fracture (with or without "bite")
    - Metacarpal shaft fracture
    - MCP joint dislocation

- **Treatment**
    - Undisplaced fractures are treated in gutter splints or casts with outriggers
    - Index and long metacarpals have limited carpometacarpal motion, requiring reduction (open or closed) with pinning if the fractures are more than 10 degrees angulated; carpometacarpal motion is greater in the ring and little metacarpals, allowing greater angulation to be accepted
    - Reduction is attempted for angulation of >30 degrees, although some surgeons accept much greater angulation for the fifth metacarpal

- **Pearl**

Angulation is important, but rotational deformity can result in significant disability and should be corrected, if present.

References

Dumont C, et al.: Clinical results of absorbable plates for displaced metacarpal fractures. J Hand Surg [Am] 2007;32:491. [PMID: 17398359]

Poolman RW, et al.: Conservative treatment for closed fifth (small finger) metacarpal neck fractures. Cochrane Database Syst Rev 2005;CD003210. [PMID: 16034891]

Finger Fractures: Proximal & Middle Phalanges

ICD-9: 816.01 Closed, middle, or proximal;
816.02 Closed, distal

- ### Essentials of Diagnosis
  - Fractures may occur at the base, neck, or shaft, or be intra-articular; also defined as open or closed
  - Many are job or sports related
  - Pain and swelling with decreased range of active motion, and possibly deformity, are reported after a history of trauma
  - Tenderness to palpation; pain with passive motion
  - Swelling and ecchymosis may be present
  - Radiographic exam is diagnostic; comparison views may be helpful if the physes are open

- ### Differential Diagnosis
  - Dislocation (proximal or distal interphalangeal joint)
  - Metacarpophalangeal (MCP) dislocation
  - Flexor tendon avulsion
  - Pathologic fracture (enchondroma)

- ### Treatment
  - Treatment can be complicated by stiffness due to adhesions of the tendons to the bony fracture callus
  - Undisplaced fractures can be treated with splinting, either a gutter splint (radial or ulnar, depending on the fracture) or a short-arm cast with an outrigger to protect the digit; splinting for 1–2 wk can be followed with buddy taping; healing occurs in 4–6 wk
  - Displaced fractures with angular, rotational, or especially intra-articular deformity require correction of the deformity with either closed reduction (with or without pinning) or open reduction and internal fixation; shortening or proximal migration of the distal fragment can also be an indication for more aggressive treatment

- ### Pearl
To avoid stiffness of the MCP joint in any hand fracture, immobilization should always place the MCP joint at 70–90 degrees of flexion ("intrinsic-plus" position).

Reference

Freeland AE, Lindley SG: Malunions of the finger metacarpals and phalanges. Hand Clin 2006;22:341. [PMID: 16843800]

9

Pediatric Problems

Physeal (Growth Plate) Fracture

ICD-9: 810–829 By location

- **Essentials of Diagnosis**

  - Salter-Harris classification: *type I*—fracture through physis; *type II*—fracture through metaphysis and physis; *type III*—fracture through epiphysis and physis; *type IV*—fracture through metaphysis into epiphysis; *type V*—crush injury to physis
  - Physeal injuries are more common than ligament injuries
  - Any growth plate can be injured; injuries most commonly occur to the distal radius, humerus, femur, tibia, and the phalanges
  - Significant injury is noted on history
  - Swelling and tenderness are noted at the physeal area
  - Types II—IV can be diagnosed by initial roentgenographic exam; types I and V frequently only demonstrate roentgenographic signs of fracture at follow-up imaging

- **Differential Diagnosis**

  - Soft tissue injury
  - Nondisplaced fracture
  - Torus or buckle fracture

- **Treatment**

  - Type I, nondisplaced type II: careful observation, closed treatment with cast or splint
  - Displaced type II: percutaneous fixation is indicated for significantly displaced fractures; it may be difficult to obtain an anatomic closed reduction in type II fractures due to interposed periosteum
  - Types III and IV: these intra-articular fractures, if displaced, require open treatment
  - Types I and V: may be difficult to see on radiographs; a high index of suspicion is necessary to warn the family of potential complications affecting the growth process

- **Pearl**

Injuries to the growth plate heal very quickly (3–4 wk); significant remodeling can occur depending on the age of the patient. Expeditious treatment is necessary to correct fracture deformity before healing takes place, if reduction is required.

Reference

Rodriguez-Merchan EC: Pediatric skeletal trauma: a review and historical perspective. Clin Orthop Relat Res 2005;432:8. [PMID: 15738799]

Supracondylar Fracture of the Humerus in Children

ICD-9: 812.41 Closed

- **Essentials of Diagnosis**
  - Most often occurs secondary to falls (extension or flexion type) or direct trauma; extension-type injury (more common) is sustained by falling onto the extended elbow and may have an intra-condylar or intracapsular aspect; flexion-type injury is a fall sustained with a flexed elbow
  - Peak ages for fracture are 5 and 8 y; right side is more common than left; equal incidence in boys and girls
  - Conduct careful physical exam distally, because such injuries are often associated with vascular and nerve damage; elbow is swollen and tender
  - Radiographs are diagnostic; comparison views to other elbow can be helpful

- **Differential Diagnosis**
  - Humeral shaft fracture
  - Intercondylar fracture of distal humerus
  - Olecranon fracture
  - Lateral condyle fracture
  - Elbow dislocation

- **Treatment**
  - In minimally displaced and stable fractures, splinting may be adequate; splinting in forearm pronation and elbow flexion is recommended
  - Percutaneous pinning is also an option for displaced fractures, enabling early flexion and extension at the elbow; pinning is also necessary if the fracture is not stable in ≤ 90 degrees of elbow flexion; immobilization in >90 degrees of flexion is associated with vascular occlusion
  - Because of the tendency for reduced, displaced fractures to redisplace, closed reduction and pinning is preferred
  - If alignment and stability is not achieved by pinning or closed reduction, perform open reduction and internal fixation

- **Pearl**

When surgical reduction is delayed >8 h, there is a greater chance that the fracture will require open reduction and pinning, as opposed to closed reduction and pinning.

References

Baratz M, et al.: Pediatric supracondylar humerus fractures. Hand Clin 2006;22:69. [PMID: 16504779]

Walmsley PJ, et al.: Delay increases the need for open reduction of type III supracondylar fractures of the humerus. J Bone Joint Surg Br 2006;88:528. [PMID: 16567791]

Osteochondritis Dissecans

ICD-9: 732.7 Site not specified

- ■ Essentials of Diagnosis
  - Poorly understood process affecting many joint surfaces (knee, capitellum, talus); trauma and ischemia probably play a role
  - Most common in children aged 8–14 y but also seen in adults
  - In the knee, most common on lateral side of medial femoral condyle
  - Symptoms are highly variable and range from vague aching after strenuous activity to pain, swelling, and possible locking or catching
  - Physical exam shows tenderness and effusion
  - Radiographs show a lesion close to the articular surface
  - MRI (± arthrogram) can delineate whether cartilage is intact over the lesion

- ■ Differential Diagnosis
  - Meniscal tear (knee)
  - Loose body
  - Osteochondral fracture

- ■ Treatment
  - Depends on patient age, size of fragment, condition of overlying cartilage, and location
  - Asymptomatic young children need no treatment
  - Older children with symptoms can be treated as adults, with immobilization or limited weight bearing for 6 wk for the knee or ankle
  - Treatment options include drilling, fixation of the fragment with bone grafting, or excision and debridement with either drilling, osteoarticular autologous transplantation (OATS), or autologous chondrocyte implantation (ACI)
  - Removal of large osteochondral fragments from the knee yields poor results

- ■ Pearl

Ossification fronts may be a normal variant and are seen bilaterally, in contrast to osteochondritis dissecans, which is typically unilateral.

References

Crawford DC, Safran MR: Osteochondritis dissecans of the knee. J Am Acad Orthop Surg 2006;14:90. [PMID: 16467184]

Yadao MA, et al.: Osteochondritis dissecans of the elbow. Instr Course Lect 2004;53:599. [PMID: 15116649]

Child Abuse

ICD-9: E967.0 Male partner; E967.1 Other person;
E967.2 Female partner

- ■ Essentials of Diagnosis
  - • Associated with young parents who have a child with special needs; only a slight association with ethnic or economic groups
  - • Key factor in diagnosis is whether the history supports the physical and radiographic findings
  - • Long bone fractures in children <2 y with a questionable history are considered abuse until proven otherwise
  - • History of delay in seeking treatment
  - • Findings may include limb deformity, swelling, ecchymosis, and multiple healing fractures of various ages seen on radiographs

- ■ Differential Diagnosis
  - • Shaken baby syndrome
  - • Bone fragility syndrome
  - • Neoplastic process

- ■ Treatment
  - • Provide pain control and fracture treatment, by casting or splinting
  - • Contact Child Protective Services in suspicious cases

- ■ Pearl

Child abuse affects a significant fraction of the population and is the leading cause of morbidity and mortality throughout childhood.

Reference

Oral R, et al.: Fractures in young children: are physicians in the emergency department and orthopedic clinics adequately screening for possible abuse. Pediatr Emerg Care 2003;19:148. [PMID: 12813297]

Torus (Buckle) Fracture

ICD-9: 813.45 Radius; 813.44 Radius and ulna;
823.4 Distal tibia

- ■ Essentials of Diagnosis
  - Typically the dorsal surface of the radius is buckled, due to a fall on an outstretched hand in a child, but any long bone can be involved; the ulna can also be involved
  - Torus (buckle) represents failure on the compression side of the bone; if failure is on the tension side of the fracture a "green-stick" fracture occurs
  - Stable and less painful than displaced fractures; often mistaken for a wrist sprain
  - Tender to palpation at the fracture site, possibly some swelling

- ■ Differential Diagnosis
  - Sprain
  - Physeal injury (Salter-Harris)
  - Buckle injury to the scaphoid

- ■ Treatment
  - Heals uneventfully in 3–4 wk; immobilization is indicated for comfort
  - A short-arm cast or splint serves well for radius-ulna fractures
  - Casting is perhaps better than splinting for less-compliant patients and may be necessary for torus fractures of the femur or tibia

- ■ Pearl

Buckle fractures may not present with the typical bulge of the cortex; instead, they may merely show a cortical angulation.

References

Plint AC, et al.: A randomized, controlled trial of removable splinting versus casting for wrist buckle fractures in children. Pediatrics 2006;117:691. [PMID: 16510648]

West S, et al.: Buckle fractures of the distal radius are safely treated in a soft bandage: a randomized prospective trial of the bandage versus plaster cast. J Pediatr Orthop 2005;25:322. [PMID: 15832147]

Amniotic Constriction Bands

ICD-9: 762.8

- Essentials of Diagnosis
  - Occur when protein-rich amniotic fluid coalesces, forming constrictive bands around the limbs of a fetus in utero
  - May cause necrosis or even amputation in utero or soon after birth
  - At birth, band is seen as a circumferential depression in the skin and soft tissues of the extremity, almost as if a wire had been tied around the limb; distally there is persistent edema
  - Occasionally bands must be released at birth to prevent necrosis distally

- Differential Diagnosis
  - None

- Treatment
  - Bands are released using Z-plasty techniques to eliminate the constriction
  - Procedure is usually staged in 2 steps, to avoid compromising the blood supply to the entire limb; one-stage release has also been described

- Pearl

Constriction bands can also be released in utero using endoscopy.

Reference

Gabos PG: Modified technique for the surgical treatment of congenital constriction bands of the arms and legs of infants and children. Orthopedics 2006;29:401. [PMID: 16729738]

Syndactyly

ICD-9: 755.11 Fingers, soft tissue; 755.12 Fingers, bone fusion; 755.13 Toes, soft tissue; 755.14 Toes, bone fusion

- **Essentials of Diagnosis**
    - Most common genetic hand deformity (1 in 2000 live births); cause is unknown; more common in Caucasians; male:female ratio is 2:1
    - Bilateral in 50% of cases
    - Two categories: simple is the joining of soft tissue of 2 or more digits; complex is the joining of soft tissue, bone, or joints of 2 or more digits
    - Complex syndactyly occurs frequently with other congenital diseases, such as Apert syndrome
    - Other abnormalities associated with syndactyly include polydactyly, cleft hands, Poland syndrome, Down syndrome, fetal hydantoin syndrome, and ring constrictions

- **Differential Diagnosis**
    - Various congenital syndromes, including Apert, Pfeiffer, and Cenani-Lenz syndactyly

- **Treatment**
    - Surgery is indicated when webbing occurs within a few millimeters distal to the point of normal separation of the fingers and affects normal function
    - Ideal age for finger release is 6–18 mo
    - Surgical procedure includes creation of a local flap and full-thickness skin graft to provide adequate surface coverage
    - Syndactyly is rarely treated in the foot

- **Pearl**

Syndactyly is a failure of apoptosis (ie, programmed cell death), which is a normal part of development.

Reference

Talamillo A, et al.: The developing limb and the control of the number of digits. Clin Genet 2005;67:143. [PMID: 15679824]

Polydactyly

ICD-9: 755.01 Fingers; 755.02 Toes

- **Essentials of Diagnosis**
  - Polydactyly, the presence of extra digits, is one of the most frequent congenital disorders and the most common limb deformity of the hand; it also frequently occurs on the foot
  - May be hereditary and bilateral; cause is unknown
  - In the US, polydactyly is more common in African Americans than in other racial and ethnic groups
  - Radial polydactyly usually causes a duplicated thumb; the ulnar thumb component is usually more developed
  - Extent of bifurcation can vary from 2 distal phalanges with 2 nails, to 2 entire thumbs
  - Radiographs are usually required to determine bone and joint involvement

- **Differential Diagnosis**
  - Meckel-Gruber syndrome (polydactyly seen on fetal ultrasound)
  - Pallister-Hall syndrome
  - Other associated syndromes (eg, Holt-Oram; Fanconi)

- **Treatment**
  - Excision of extra digit(s) at 6–12 mo when on the ulnar side of the hand
  - For radial digits, merging of the elements of both digits (usually keeping the ulnar thumb) is necessary to obtain optimal function of the reconstructed digit

- **Pearl**

Preaxial (radial digits and medial toes) and postaxial (ulnar digits and lateral toes) polydactyly often accompanies genetic syndromes and should prompt the physician to look for other problems (renal, cardiac, etc).

References

Schwabe GC, Mundlos S: Genetics of congenital hand anomalies. Handchir Mikrochir Plast Chir 2004;36:85. [PMID: 15162306]

Talamillo A, et al.: The developing limb and the control of the number of digits. Clin Genet 2005;67:143. [PMID: 15679824]

In-Toeing in Children

ICD-9: 754.53 Metatarsus adductus; 736.89 Internal tibial torsion; 755.60 Femoral anteversion

- Essentials of Diagnosis
  - In-toeing can present in early to mid-childhood; patient is usually <5 y of age with a complaint of "pigeon-toe" gait
  - Internal rotation of the foot can occur due to rotation of the foot, tibia, or femur from metatarsus adductus (MA), internal tibial torsion (ITT), or femoral anteversion (FA)
  - MA resolves by ~1 y; femur and tibia are normal in alignment, and hip is normal (see also Metatarsus Adductus)
  - ITT resolves at age 3–4 y; patella points forward but foot and ankle are internally rotated (lateral malleolus is *not* posterior to medial malleolus, as is normal), and hip version is normal (see also Internal Tibial Torsion)
  - FA resolves by ~10 y; foot and tibia are normal but on standing, patellae try to "kiss" each other (ie, are internally rotated); hip has more internal rotation than external rotation; femur must internally rotate to keep femoral head covered by acetabulum, and foot goes with rest of leg (see also Femoral Anteversion, Increased)
  - Radiographs are normal

- Differential Diagnosis
  - Bowlegs (genu varum)
  - Blount disease
  - Osteogenesis imperfecta
  - Trauma
  - Rickets
  - Neurofibromatosis

- Treatment
  - Significant asymmetry is cause for concern; otherwise, observation and reassurance is indicated
  - Spontaneous resolution is expected, as these are physiologic variations of normal anatomy

- Pearl

Often the most difficult part of reassuring parents is convincing a grandmother that the child does not need braces, because historically, these physiologic conditions were often treated with bracing. Six-month follow-up with careful exams to point out improvement is helpful.

Reference

Lincoln TL, Suen PW: Common rotational variations in children. J Am Acad Orthop Surg 2003;11:312. [PMID: 14565753]

Metatarsus Adductus

ICD-9: 754.53

- ■ Essentials of Diagnosis
  - • Most common foot deformity in the newborn; may be unilateral
  - • May cause apparent in-toeing in children
  - • Forefoot is held in adduction and inversion, usually mild and flexible; hindfoot is normal
  - • In severe cases, an oblique groove is noted on the medial side of the foot

- ■ Differential Diagnosis
  - • Internal tibial torsion
  - • Clubfoot
  - • Metatarsus primus varus
  - • Cerebral palsy

- ■ Treatment
  - • Generally no treatment is needed as the condition frequently resolves by 12–18 mo of age
  - • Stretching exercises and, in resistant cases, short-leg casting will accomplish correction
  - • Surgical release is necessary for older children with residual metatarsus adductus and pain or trouble fitting shoes; medial capsulotomy and abductor hallucis lengthening are performed

- ■ Pearl

Typical metatarsus adductus tends to be self-correcting with the weight bearing of walking.

Reference

Lincoln TL, Suen PW: Common rotational variations in children. J Am Acad Orthop Surg 2003;11:312. [PMID: 14565753]

Internal Tibial Torsion

ICD-9: 736.89

- Essentials of Diagnosis
  - Internal tibial torsion is the most common cause of in-toeing in children <2 y
  - At birth, torsion is usually bilateral, familial, and as high as 30–40 degrees
  - Tibial torsion can be measured either by the prone thigh-foot angle, or by comparing the plane of the patella to the bimalleolar axis
  - Radiographic assessment is of no value

- Differential Diagnosis
  - Femoral anteversion
  - Metatarsus adductus
  - Clubfoot (talipes equinovarus)

- Treatment
  - Clinical monitoring; bracing is ineffective
  - Spontaneous resolution with normal growth and development can be anticipated
  - Improvement usually does not occur until the child begins to stand and walk
  - Full resolution may not occur until 4 y of age

- Pearl

Rarely, persistent internal tibial torsion in an older child or adolescent may require surgical derotation.

References

Accadbled F, Cahuzac JP: ["In-toeing and out-toeing."] Rev Prat 2006;56:165. [PMID: 16584043]

Lincoln TL, Suen PW: Common rotational variations in children. J Am Acad Orthop Surg 2003;11:312. [PMID: 14565753]

Femoral Anteversion, Increased

ICD-9: 755.60

- **Essentials of Diagnosis**
  - Femoral torsion (version) is the angular difference between the femoral neck axis and the transcondylar axis of the knee; the femoral head and neck almost always point anterior to the transcondylar axis (anteversion) as compared to retroversion
  - Neonates have as much as 40 degrees of femoral anteversion; by age 8–9 y, average anteversion has decreased to the typical adult value of 15 degrees
  - Regression of anteversion can be delayed or incomplete, resulting in excessive—or excessive for age—anteversion
  - Femoral anteversion is the most common cause of in-toeing in early childhood, and the child is usually brought to the physician's attention by a complaint of in-toeing
  - Child sits in the "W" position with knees internally rotated and adducted and runs in an "eggbeater" fashion
  - Physical exam shows limited external rotation of the hip compared with internal rotation
  - CT scan is required for accurate evaluation of femoral torsion

- **Differential Diagnosis**
  - Internal tibial torsion
  - Metatarsus adductus

- **Treatment**
  - Observation is indicated; orthoses are not effective
  - Surgery is indicated in children >8 or 9 y with residual cosmetic or functional deformity (anteversion >50 degrees, internal hip rotation >80 degrees)

- **Pearl**

If concomitant with external tibial torsion, femoral anteversion is associated with increased knee pain.

Reference

Lincoln TL, Suen PW: Common rotational variations in children. J Am Acad Orthop Surg 2003;11:312. [PMID: 14565753]

Tarsal Coalition

ICD-9: 755.67

- **Essentials of Diagnosis**
  - Congenital connection between 2 or more tarsal bones; autosomal-dominant inheritance; bilateral in 50% of cases
  - Presents in adolescence as coalitions become increasingly ossified; often preceded by sprains and other minor injuries
  - Also called *peroneal spastic flatfoot* because peroneus longus and brevis become protectively overactive
  - Produces significant decrease in transverse tarsal motion and tenderness over the sinus tarsi; fixed valgus of heel
  - Talocalcaneal coalition (medial facet) causes constant activity-related pain, significant reduction in subtalar motion, and tender medial subtalar joint; calcaneonavicular coalition (most common coalition) causes intermittent symptoms, little reduction in subtalar motion
  - Diagnosis: CT scan, also seen on AP and lateral radiographs
  - Lateral view shows talar beaking, indicating traction spur on superior surface of talar head; C sign (bean-shaped density coincides with bridging in region of sustentaculum tali); anteater nose sign of calcaneonavicular coalition (anterior process of calcaneus extends beyond calcaneocuboid joint)

- **Differential Diagnosis**
  - Inflammation (osteochondroses, juvenile rheumatoid arthritis)
  - Infection
  - Tumor (osteoid osteoma)
  - Trauma

- **Treatment**
  - Decreased activity, orthosis, medication, and casting
  - Calcaneonavicular coalition may require excision of coalition with interposition of extensor brevis; talocalcaneal coalition requires resection and interposition of fat if condition involves < 50% of subtalar joint
  - Hindfoot fusion or triple arthrodesis in late or neglected cases to alleviate pain and deformity

- **Pearl**

Consider this diagnosis in children with frequent ankle sprains. Lack of normal subtalar and transverse tarsal motion causes pronation and supination of the foot through the ankle joint.

References

Bohne WH: Tarsal coalition. Curr Opin Pediatr 2001;13:29. [PMID: 11176240]
Crim JR, Kjeldsberg KM: Radiographic diagnosis of tarsal coalition. AJR Am J Roentgenol 2004;182:323. [PMID: 14736655]

Calcaneovalgus Foot

ICD-9: 754.62 Talipes calcaneovalgus;
755.69 Congenital deformity of ankle

- ■ Essentials of Diagnosis
  - Birth abnormality caused by intrauterine positioning in which the hindfoot is markedly dorsiflexed, everted, and abducted and rests against the anterior tibia
  - Physical exam shows limited range of motion, with plantar flexion limited to 90 degrees

- ■ Differential Diagnosis
  - Congenital vertical talus
  - Oblique talus, talonavicular subluxation
  - Paralytic pes valgus

- ■ Treatment
  - Abnormal foot position resolves spontaneously by 2–3 mo
  - Consider passive stretching exercises versus bracing, casting if refractory

- ■ Pearl

All true calcaneovalgus feet resolve spontaneously by 2–3 mo.

Reference

Furdon SA, Donlon CR: Examination of the newborn foot: positional and structural abnormalities. Adv Neonatal Care 2002;2:248. [PMID: 12881938]

Congenital Clubfoot

ICD-9: 754.51

- Essentials of Diagnosis
  - Congenital, fixed deformity of the foot characterized by plantar flexion (equinus), inversion, axial internal rotation of subtalar joint (varus), and medial subluxation of talonavicular and calcaneocuboid joints (adductus); also called *talipes equinovarus*
  - Occurs 1 in 1000 births, more commonly in males; polygenic inheritance pattern; bilateral in 50% of cases
  - Always associated with a decrease in calf circumference related to muscle fibrosis; to rule out presence of an associated spinal deformity, observe for caudal dimpling, hairy patches, or other associated findings
  - Often diagnosed prenatally with ultrasound
  - In infants, radiographs are usually unnecessary because foot bones have not ossified; radiographs may be taken when the child presents at walking age; anterior talocalcaneal angle is reduced (normal = 30–55 degrees) on AP view; talocalcaneal angle is reduced (normal = 25–50 degrees) on lateral view

- Differential Diagnosis
  - Myotonic muscular dystrophy
  - Poliomyelitis
  - Cerebral palsy
  - Metatarsus adductus
  - Spinal deformities with neurologic sequelae (eg, spina bifida, myelomeningocele)

- Treatment
  - Serial manipulation and casting is first-line treatment; initially, casts are molded to correct cavus deformity, followed by correction of forefoot adduction and heel varus, and, finally, correction of equinus (Ponseti technique); if casting is unsuccessful after ~12 wk, consider operative correction
  - Mild recurrence is fairly common; advise parents that fully corrected foot will have some residual stiffness, calf size will remain small, and foot will be smaller than contralateral foot

- Pearl

Casting should begin immediately after birth to take advantage of initial elasticity of contracted ligaments.

References

Roye DP Jr, Roye BD: Idiopathic congenital talipes equinovarus. J Am Acad Orthop Surg 2002;10:239. [PMID: 15089073]

Scher DM: The Ponseti method for treatment of congenital club foot. Curr Opin Pediatr 2006;18:22. [PMID: 16470157]

Congenital Flatfoot

ICD-9: 754.61

- ■ Essentials of Diagnosis
  - Also called *pes planus*; flexible flatfoot (the predominant cause of congenital flatfoot) is present from birth but is often not recognized until the end of the first or during the second decade of life
  - Condition probably represents a normal variant of the longitudinal arch and usually is asymptomatic
  - Always symmetric (bilateral) and passively correctable when the foot is examined in the suspended position
  - Achilles tendon contracture and equinus deformity are usually not present
  - Radiographic standing lateral view shows sagging of talometatarsal angle, which is normally 0 degrees; an angle of 0–15 degrees represents mild flatfoot; 15–30 is moderate; and >30, severe
  - Adolescents and adults with congenital flatfoot are susceptible to posterior tibialis tendonitis

- ■ Differential Diagnosis
  - Symptomatic flexible flatfoot
  - Tarsal coalition
  - Flatfoot associated with an accessory navicular
  - Marfan syndrome
  - Ehlers-Danlos syndrome

- ■ Treatment
  - Longitudinal arch support may benefit patients with mild symptoms of flexible flatfoot; Achilles strengthening exercises may also help
  - Patients with symptomatic flexible flatfoot who have not responded to conservative treatment may respond to a calcaneal lengthening osteotomy (Evans procedure)

- ■ Pearl

Surgery is never necessary for asymptomatic flatfoot.

Reference

Dockery GL: Symptomatic juvenile flatfoot condition: surgical treatment. J Foot Ankle Surg 1995;34:135. [PMID: 7599611]

Congenital Vertical Talus

ICD-9: 754.61

- ■ Essentials of Diagnosis
  - Rare condition, present at birth; basically a dorsal dislocation of the forefoot; also known as *rockerbottom foot*
  - More than 80% of cases are associated with other syndromes and anomalies (eg, Marfan syndrome, arthrogryposis, myelomeningocele, etc)
  - Continuum from relatively mild to severe; may be unilateral but frequently is bilateral
  - Foot appears to have a "rocker" bottom on exam; heel is in rigid valgus
  - On lateral radiographs, the talus is vertical, hence the name; radiographs are diagnostic

- ■ Differential Diagnosis
  - Calcaneovalgus flatfoot
  - Various other syndromes (myelodysplasia; arthrogryposis; trisomies 13, 14, 15, and 18)

- ■ Treatment
  - Treatment has traditionally been casting, followed by extensive surgical releases, because the disorder is resistant to conservative treatment
  - For patients who are nonambulatory, shoe modifications can be used to protect the foot
  - Recently, closed management with casts and pinning with Achilles tenotomy have been reported to be successful

- ■ Pearl

Unless the cause of the vertical talus is clear, the patient should have a complete genetic and neuromuscular workup.

Reference

Dobbs MB, et al.: Early results of a new method of treatment for idiopathic congenital vertical talus. J Bone Joint Surg Am 2006;88:1192. [PMID: 16757750]

Adolescent Bunions (Hallux Valgus)

ICD-9: 754.52, 755.66

- **Essentials of Diagnosis**
  - Differs from adult form in that a medial-sided bunion may not always be present, widened intermetatarsal angles are almost always present, family history is positive in up to 75% of cases, and osteotomies of the metatarsal are almost always needed to obtain correction
  - As in adult form, the disorder is characterized by metatarsophalangeal (MTP) angles >15 degrees and intermetatarsal angles >9 degrees
  - Physical exam shows widened forefoot and pain over first MTP

- **Differential Diagnosis**
  - Metatarsalgia

- **Treatment**
  - Indications for surgical correction are not clearly defined; controversy remains as to whether surgical correction should be performed before or after the physes close
  - Pain and difficulty with shoe wearing are good indications for surgery; an unattractive, progressive deformity in a patient with a positive family history may also be an indication for surgery
  - Distal metatarsal "Chevron" osteotomies may be performed for hallux valgus angles of up to 30 degrees and intermetatarsal angles of up to 30 degrees, whereas proximal metatarsal osteotomies should be performed for larger deformities

- **Pearl**

Recurrence of the deformity is more common in the adolescent form than the adult form.

Reference

Johnson AE, et al.: Treatment of adolescent hallux valgus with the first metatarsal double osteotomy: the denver experience. J Pediatr Ortho 2004;24:358. [PMID: 15205615]

Bowlegs (Genu Varum) & Knock-Knees (Genu Valgum) in Children

ICD-9: 755.64 Genu varum; 755.69 Genu valgum

■ Essentials of Diagnosis

- Children aged 0–2 y may have physiologic, bilateral, symmetric bowing of legs (physiologic genu varum); normal is 10–15 degrees; maximum deformity at 18 mo
- Children aged 3–6 y may show exaggerated knock-kneed condition (physiologic genu valgum), up to 15 degrees of valgus may be normal; maximum deformity at 3–3.5 y
- Radiographs show symmetric flaring of tibia and femur

■ Differential Diagnosis

- Genu varum: Blount disease, internal tibial torsion, osteogenesis imperfecta, osteochondroma, trauma, dysplasia, rickets
- Genu valgum: renal osteodystrophy, tumor (osteochondroma, Ollier disease), infection, trauma (physeal injury), fibrous dysplasia, neurofibromatosis

■ Treatment

- Leg bowing in infants and excessive knock-knees in 6-y-olds are normal phenomena; observe
- Asymmetric bowing or knock-knee is not normal and deserves further evaluation
- Genu varum that progresses shows >50% of the deformity on the tibia in almost all patients
- Bowing that persists beyond 3 y of age requires further evaluation; rule out structural abnormality
- Internal tibial torsion spontaneously resolves by age 4 y
- Consider surgery (hemiepiphysiodesis, physeal stapling) for genu valgum in children >10 y with >10 cm between medial malleoli or >15–20 degrees of valgus

■ Pearl

Internal tibial torsion can masquerade as bowing of knees when the child walks with feet forward as knees are then rotated externally.

References

Bowen RE, et al.: Relative tibial and femoral varus as a predictor of progression of varus deformities of the lower limbs in young children. J Pediatr Orthop 2002;22:105. [PMID: 11744864]

Gordon JE, et al.: Femoral deformity in tibia vara. J Bone Joint Surg Am 2006;88:380. [PMID: 16452751]

Blount Disease

ICD-9: 736.42

- **Essentials of Diagnosis**
  - Also called *tibia vara*, due to loss of growth on the medial tibial physis; this causes medial angulation and internal rotation of the proximal tibia
  - Infantile (0–4 y) more common; bilateral in 80% of cases; associated with obesity, female sex, African American descent
  - Gait characterized by painless varus thrust in stance phase; metaphyseal beaking; Drennan angle (metaphyseal-diaphyseal angle) >11 degrees

- **Differential Diagnosis**
  - Osteogenesis imperfecta
  - Osteochondromas
  - Rickets
  - Achondroplasia
  - Physiologic genu varum
  - Neurofibromatosis

- **Treatment**
  - Mild cases may spontaneously improve
  - Bracing for metaphyseal-diaphyseal angles of 10–15 degrees consists of a knee-ankle-foot orthosis with a single medial upright and no knee hinge; maximum trial of bracing is 1 y, but there is no consensus regarding efficacy
  - Surgery is indicated for patients with lack of correction after 1 y of bracing, physeal closure, or severe deformity
  - Corrective tibial osteotomy is performed prior to physeal closure to restore normal valgus angulation of knee
  - If deformity recurs, indicating physeal bridge formation, consider physeal bridge resection, interpositional graft, intraepiphyseal osteotomy, elevation of medial tibial plateau, and physeal excision

- **Pearl**

Once physeal bridging occurs, there is little alternative to repeated surgical correction of the angular deformity.

References

Accadbled F, et al.: One-step treatment for evolved Blount's disease: four cases and review of the literature. J Pediatr Orthop 2003;23:747. [PMID: 14581778]

Cheema JI, et al.: Radiographic characteristics of lower-extremity bowing in children. Radiographics 2003;23:871. [PMID: 12853662]

Gordon JE, et al.: Femoral deformity in tibia vara. J Bone Joint Surg Am 2006;88:380. [PMID: 16452751]

Osgood-Schlatter Disease

ICD-9: 732.4

- Essentials of Diagnosis
  - The portion of the proximal tibial epiphysis that contains the patellar tendon may experience excessive stress, causing an apophysitis; it then may enlarge in size and develop a bursa
  - Later in the disease, the apophysis may undergo fragmentation
  - History of mild to moderate pain, especially with activity; patient may complain of a "bump" on the leg
  - Physical exam shows a prominent tibial tubercle, possibly some tenderness to palpation
  - Activities to the limits of pain have no harmful effect

- Differential Diagnosis
  - Neoplasm
  - Pes anserinus bursitis
  - Avulsion of the tibial tubercle
  - Sindig-Larsen-Johansson apophysitis

- Treatment
  - Treatment includes activity modification to limit the pain
  - Quadriceps stretching is helpful and, in severe cases, casting or splinting for short periods for pain relief may be beneficial
  - Knee pads can be used for kneeling activities
  - Chopat strap can give symptomatic relief

- Pearl

Patients who develop fragmentation of the patellar apophysis have a propensity to have symptomatic patellar tendonitis into adulthood.

Reference

Cassas KJ, Cassettari-Wayhs A: Childhood and adolescent sports-related overuse injuries. Am Fam Physician 2006;73:1014. [PMID: 16570735]

Discoid Meniscus

ICD-9: 717.5

- ■ Essentials of Diagnosis
  - During early embryologic development, the knee menisci are discoid in shape; normally, during development in utero, they gradually become semilunar
  - If the lateral meniscus does not become semilunar and remains discoid, its ability to cup the lateral femoral condyle is reduced, which may cause instability of the knee or hypermobility of the discoid meniscus
  - Three types of discoid meniscus: complete, incomplete, and Wrisberg (in which the posterior portion of the meniscus is not attached, resulting in a hypermobile meniscus)
  - Children >10 y with this condition are susceptible to tears of the meniscus
  - Pain may be a presenting complaint
  - A click is heard over the lateral knee with flexion and extension; occasionally an effusion is present
  - Radiographs may reveal slight lateral joint space widening; MRI is diagnostic

- ■ Differential Diagnosis
  - Lateral meniscus tear
  - Iliotibial band syndrome

- ■ Treatment
  - Asymptomatic discoid menisci are not treated; if the discoid meniscus is stable at the rim and symptomatic, arthroscopic saucerization of the middle of the meniscus is performed
  - Meniscal repair of unstable menisci is recommended to prevent secondary osteoarthritis

- ■ Pearl

Total excision of the discoid lateral meniscus leads to osteoarthritis.

Reference

Kelly BT, Green DW: Discoid lateral meniscus in children. Curr Opin Pediatr 2002;14:54. [PMID: 11880735]

Cerebral Palsy: Pediatric

ICD-9: 343.9

- Essentials of Diagnosis
  - Static encephalopathy that occurs in prenatal or perinatal period; key component is increased muscle tone, either spasticity (increased tone with stretch) or dystonia (increased tone without stretch)
  - Four anatomic patterns: (1) *hemiplegia*—involves one side of body; often caused by congenital loss of parietal or cerebral cortex; intelligence and development are often normal; (2) *diplegia*—often associated with prematurity or intracerebral hemorrhage; typically produces symmetric involvement of lower and upper extremities (but often less severe in upper); child often has normal intelligence but developmental delays; (3) *quadriplegia*—causes severe spasticity, mental retardation, joint contractures, seizures; most common with birth asphyxia or encephalitis; (4) *mixed neurologic involvement*—athetosis, ballismus, ataxia in addition to spasticity

- Differential Diagnosis
  - Arthrogryposis
  - Myelomeningocele
  - Familial spastic paraparesis
  - Nonstatic encephalopathy (ongoing metabolic, infectious, or ischemic insult)
  - Toxicities (lead poisoning)

- Treatment
  - Requires coordinated treatment effort of providers and parents
  - PT and OT may be beneficial early in life and after surgical releases; bracing often helps control spasticity and decrease deformity; medication (eg, oral baclofen) and botulinum toxin or phenol injections can also help decrease spasticity
  - Surgery (adductor release; Achilles, hamstring, gastrocnemius, or iliopsoas lengthening) can help control spasticity; reconstructive surgery is used to correct hip subluxation or dislocation and scoliosis

- Pearl

Upper extremity surgery is most beneficial for patients with normal intelligence, good body posture, and voluntary control of movements (ie, nonathetoid cerebral palsy).

References

Koman LA, et al.: Cerebral palsy. Lancet 2004;363:1619. [PMID: 15145637]

Paneth N, et al.: The descriptive epidemiology of cerebral palsy. Clin Perinatol 2006;33:251. [PMID: 16765723]

Spinal Muscular Atrophy

ICD-9: 335.1

- ■ Essentials of Diagnosis
  - • Autosomal-recessive genetic disorder characterized by progressive muscle weakness and hypotonia; male:female ratio is 2:1
  - • Muscle weakness is caused by degeneration of alpha motor neurons in anterior horn cells of the spinal cord, affecting proximal muscles more than distal ones
  - • Prenatal diagnosis through DNA analysis for the detection of a missing chromosome arm 5q is available
  - • Common medical complications include recurrent respiratory system infections

- ■ Differential Diagnosis
  - • Cerebral palsy
  - • Polymyositis
  - • Inflammatory myopathy
  - • Juvenile myasthenia gravis
  - • Chronic inflammatory demyelinated polyneuropathy
  - • Progressive muscular dystrophy

- ■ Treatment
  - • Most children do not require orthopaedic intervention; some may require physical therapy for prevention of contractures
  - • Surgical intervention may be utilized to treat contractures

- ■ Pearl

Spinal muscular atrophy is the most common diagnosis in young girls with progressive muscle weakness.

References

Monani UR: Spinal muscular atrophy: a deficiency in a ubiquitous protein; a motor neuron-specific disease. Neuron 2005;48:885. [PMID: 16364894]

Sumner CJ: Therapeutics development for spinal muscular atrophy. Neuro Rx 2006;3:235. [PMID: 16554261]

Arthrogryposis

ICD-9: 728.3, 754.89

- Essentials of Diagnosis
  - Arthrogryposis multiplex congenita ("multiple congenital contractures") is a rare autosomal-recessive disorder characterized by deformed, rigid joints and muscle atrophy
  - Many cases are neurogenic in origin (can involve myogenic, skeletal, or environmental factors)
  - Involved extremities are cylindrical, fusiform, or cone shaped
  - Dislocation of joints, rigid skeletal deformities (eg, clubfoot), and shiny skin with decreased wrinkling are characteristic clinical features

- Differential Diagnosis
  - Myelomeningocele
  - Moebius syndrome
  - Larson syndrome
  - Clubfoot (talipes equinovarus)
  - Congenital myasthenia gravis
  - Bruck syndrome

- Treatment
  - Includes passive stretching exercises for each contracted joint, with splinting
  - Osteotomies are often required to correct deformities or transfer range of motion to a more useful arc (near skeletal maturity)
  - Other surgical approaches include tenotomies with capsulotomy and capsulectomy with casting; correction should be obtained at time of surgery
  - Clubfeet require surgical correction

- Pearl

Sensation and intellect are normal.

References

Beals RK: The distal arthrogryposes: a new classification of peripheral contractures. Clin Orthop Relat Res 2005;203. [PMID: 15930940]

Mennen U, et al.: Arthrogryposis multiplex congenita. J Hand Surg [Br] 2005;30:468. [PMID: 16061316]

Congenital Posteromedial Bowing of the Tibia

ICD-9: 754.43

- ■ Essentials of Diagnosis
  - • Unilateral birth deformity of distal one quarter of the tibia; not associated with other congenital deformities
  - • Apex of the bow is posteromedial (usually ~50 degrees) and often has an associated overlying skin dimple
  - • Spatial orientation of the ankle, not the foot, is responsible for the deformity
  - • Clinical findings include posteromedial bowing of the distal tibia, limb-length discrepancy (usually 1–1.5 cm at birth), and triceps surae weakness
  - • Important to differentiate from *anterolateral bowing* of the tibia, which occurs from pseudoarthrosis and *does not* spontaneously resolve

- ■ Differential Diagnosis
  - • Calcaneovalgus foot
  - • Congenital pseudoarthrosis of the tibia

- ■ Treatment
  - • Despite its dramatic appearance, congenital posteromedial bowing of the tibia resolves spontaneously in all cases
  - • Casting of the foot or ankle has no role nor offers any advantage toward recovery
  - • Tibial curve usually resolves enough clinically so that by age 2 y the limb appears straight, although bowing may be seen radiographically until the age of 5–8 y
  - • All patients will have a residual limb-length discrepancy that is proportional to the amount of shortening apparent at birth (affected side is shorter); this discrepancy (often ~4 cm at maturity) will require follow-up and appropriate treatment, including ipsilateral limb lengthening and contralateral epiphysiodesis

- ■ Pearl

Although alignment corrects spontaneously, limb-length discrepancy and some muscle atrophy persist.

References

Cheema JI, et al.: Radiographic characteristics of lower-extremity bowing in children. Radiographics 2003;23:871. [PMID: 12853662]

Pappas AM: Congenital posteromedial bowing of the tibia and fibula. J Pediatr Orthop 1984;4:525. [PMID: 6490868]

Congenital Pseudarthrosis of the Tibia

ICD-9: 755.69 Congenital angulation of tibia;
733.16 Pathologic fracture; 733.82 Pseudarthrosis

- Essentials of Diagnosis
  - Bowing of the tibia at birth is a harbinger of congenital pseudarthrosis of the tibia (CPT); etiology is unknown
  - Apex of the bow is anterolateral (opposite of posteromedial bowing, which is benign and often has an associated overlying skin dimple)
  - Left side is affected to a greater degree than right
  - Associated with neurofibromatosis in 40–80% of cases
  - Radiographs prior to fracture shows sclerosis at the area of bowing

- Differential Diagnosis
  - Anterolateral tibial bowing with duplication of the hallux
  - Paraxial tibial hemimelia
  - Paraxial fibular hemimelia

- Treatment
  - Patients with bowing but no fracture are best treated with a total contact orthosis to prevent fracture and pseudarthrosis
  - Casting of the leg after fracture has occurred is appropriate until a pseudarthrosis is apparent; pseudarthrosis is the indication for surgery
  - Several surgical options for CPT are available, including bone grafting, internal fixation, electrical stimulation, microvascular grafts, Ilizarov fixators, and amputation; recent reports have demonstrated success with excision of the pseudarthrosis, bone grafting, and rodding
  - Most patients will have a residual limb-length discrepancy (affected side is shorter)

- Pearl

CPT is a difficult problem that will affect patients for much of their lives.

Reference

Dobbs MB, et al.: Use of an intramedullary rod for the treatment of congenital pseudarthrosis of the tibia. Surgical technique. J Bone Joint Surg Am 2005;87:33. [PMID: 15743845]

Idiopathic Scoliosis in Adolescents

ICD-9: 733.30

- ■ Essentials of Diagnosis
  - Idiopathic scoliosis is a diagnosis of exclusion; congenital (bony), myopathic, and neuropathic scoliosis, and neurofibromatosis are several other causes
  - More common in females (hereditary predisposition); right thoracic curves are more common, followed by double major (right thoracic and left lumbar) curves
  - Findings include shoulder elevation, waistline asymmetry, rib rotational deformity (rib hump) apparent on forward bending, trunk shift (upper body not centered over sacrum), and limb-length inequality
  - Neurologic exam is usually normal
  - Diagnosis is made with standing AP radiographs of the entire spine, which exclude congenital scoliosis

- ■ Differential Diagnosis
  - Leg-length discrepancy
  - Spinal cord or spine tumor
  - Proprioception disorder
  - Neuromuscular scoliosis
  - Congenital (bony) scoliosis
  - Neurofibromatosis

- ■ Treatment
  - In adolescents, observation, bracing, and surgical intervention, when indicated, are the mainstays of treatment
  - Curves with a Cobb angle <20 degrees can be observed
  - Bracing has a significant role in curves >20 degrees and <40 degrees because there is growth potential; bracing can prevent progression but will not reduce the magnitude of the deformity; many clinicians recommend the brace be worn 23 h/day, but in adolescents, compliance is an issue; bracing is continued until skeletal maturity is attained, when curves stabilize
  - Surgical fusion is considered for curves >40 degrees, which are difficult to control with braces

- ■ Pearl

Abnormal neurologic exam, atypical curve patterns, or rapidly progressive curves suggest that idiopathic scoliosis is not the diagnosis and further imaging and workup are required.

Reference

Shindle MK, et al.: Adolescent idiopathic scoliosis: modern management guidelines. J Surg Orthop Adv. 2006;15:43. [PMID: 16603112]

Limb-Length Inequality

ICD-9: 736.81

■ Essentials of Diagnosis

- May be a result of congenital deficiency or a variety of acquired conditions
- Upper extremity limb-length inequalities are usually only cosmetically problematic; lower extremity inequalities, when severe, result in functional difficulties
- Leg-length discrepancy of 1 inch (2.5 cm) is the approximate limit to tolerated inequality
- Obtain standing full lower extremity radiographs and scanograms

■ Differential Diagnosis

- Infection (osteomyelitis, septic arthritis)
- Trauma (physeal injuries)
- Poliomyelitis
- Cerebral palsy
- Neoplasm (eg, arteriovenous malformations)

■ Treatment

- Leg-length discrepancies <2.5 cm usually can be treated with a heel or shoe lift
- When limb-length inequality is recognized early, careful observation of growth rates and skeletal age of the growing child allows surgical epiphysiodesis (obliteration of the physis) on the "good" limb to stop growth; this allows the limbs to equilibrate when growth maturity is reached but has the disadvantage of reducing the final stature of the fully grown adult
- Lengthening procedures can be performed in cases of severe shortening

■ Pearl

Average rate of growth of the distal femur is 10–12 mm/y and 5–6 mm/y in the proximal tibia.

References

Jeong C, et al.: Knee arthritis in congenital short femur after Wagner lengthening. Clin Orthop 2006;451:177. [PMID: 16801863]

Vitale MA, et al.: The effect of limb length discrepancy on health-related quality of life: is the '2 cm rule' appropriate? J Pediatr Orthop B 2006;15:1. [PMID: 16280711]

Diskitis in Children

*ICD-9: 722.90; 722.91 Cervical; 722.92 Thoracic;
722.93 Lumbar*

- ■ Essentials of Diagnosis
  - Low-grade inflammatory process involving the intervertebral disk, usually in the lumbar spine
  - Children can be affected at any age but most commonly between 2 and 6 y
  - Hematogenous bacterial seeding of the disk occurs, most often from *Staphylococcus aureus*
  - Most patients refuse to walk because of pain
  - Small children may have only limited hyperextension of the spine; older children may have tenderness to palpation, pain with percussion, or paraspinal muscle spasm
  - ESR and CRP may be elevated
  - Radiographs may be normal, especially early in the course; bone scan will be positive; MRI may be helpful

- ■ Differential Diagnosis
  - Osteomyelitis in the pelvis or lower extremity
  - Septic joint in the lower extremity
  - Osteomyelitis of the vertebra
  - Malignancy

- ■ Treatment
  - If diskitis is suspected, blood cultures may be helpful
  - Disk aspiration is indicated in septic children if infection can be localized
  - If culture is not obtained, treat with empiric antistaphylococcal antibiotics for 6 wk
  - A spica cast may be beneficial for pain relief
  - Result is usually favorable and disk recovers by 3 y, if spontaneous fusion does not intervene

- ■ Pearl

Early in the disease the child may demonstrate Gower sign (using the hands to "walk up" the thighs when rising) to alleviate the pain associated with motion of the lumbar spine.

References

Brown R, et al.: Discitis in young children. J Bone Joint Surg Br 2001;83:106. [PMID: 11245515]

Karabouta Z, et al.: Discitis in toddlers: a case series and review. Acta Pediatr 2005;94:1516. [PMID: 16263635]

Slipped Capital Femoral Epiphysis (SCFE)

ICD-9: 732.2

- **Essentials of Diagnosis**
  - Hip disorder involving displacement of the femoral epiphysis posterior and medial to the neck of the femur; incidence is 10 per 100,000 in the US; peak onset is age 11–13 y (males and females); 30% of cases are bilateral
  - Can be acute (painful, prevents walking), chronic (over several months), or acute on chronic
  - Severity: mild, <25%; moderate, 25–50%; severe, >50%
  - Typical patient is overweight and in early prepuberty
  - Complaint of painful limp for ~1–3 mo; pain in thigh or groin, occasionally in the knee
  - Evaluation of the hip is necessary in any child aged 9–15 y with knee pain; children with SCFE have loss of internal rotation of hip and obligatory external rotation with flexion of the hip (diagnostic)
  - Radiographs are diagnostic in most cases; frog lateral view is most helpful because the slip is always posterior
  - If a Klein line drawn along the lateral femoral neck (AP view) or anterior femoral neck (lateral view) does not intersect any portion of the epiphysis, the child has SCFE

- **Differential Diagnosis**
  - Femoral neck fracture
  - Neoplasm
  - Knee pathology

- **Treatment**
  - Consists of pinning the hip *in situ* with 1–2 pins
  - Reduction of the slip, even in acute SCFE, risks causing avascular necrosis of the epiphysis; another complication, which may be iatrogenic from pin penetration, is chondrolysis of the articular surfaces—the higher the degree of slip, the earlier osteoarthritis will develop
  - Most cases are idiopathic, but endocrine abnormalities should be considered (ie, hypothyroidism)

- **Pearl**

A Klein line drawn on a lateral view radiograph is more sensitive in picking up subtle SCFE because the epiphysis always slips posteriorly and may not slip medially.

Reference

Aronsson DD, et al.: Slipped capital femoral epiphysis: current concepts. J Am Acad Orthop Surg 2006;14:666. [PMID: 17077339]

Legg-Calvé-Perthes Disease

ICD-9: 732.1

- ■ Essentials of Diagnosis
  - Avascular necrosis of the hip in children aged 4–10 y
  - More common in males than females; self-limited and usually unilateral
  - Affected children are usually small for age
  - Child usually presents with a painless limp; if pain is present, it may be referred to the thigh or knee
  - Physical exam shows hip flexion contracture of 0–30 degrees, with decreased abduction and internal rotation
  - Radiographs are normal early in the disease course, with progressive fragmentation, irregularity, and eventual collapse of the femoral head
  - Bone scans and MRIs are of little value

- ■ Differential Diagnosis
  - Gaucher disease (with bilateral Legg-Calvé-Perthes disease)
  - Multiple epiphyseal dysplasia

- ■ Treatment
  - Children with bone age <5 y and minor involvement do not need treatment
  - Bracing or surgery is recommended for older children and those with more advanced disease
  - Poor prognostic signs are age ≥8 y, abduction <15 degrees (stiffness), >50% of head involvements, and subluxation or lateral calcification
  - Treatment has no effect on outcome if patient has a chronologic age ≥8 y at onset of the disease

- ■ Pearl

Some evidence suggests that avascular necrosis may be a result of thrombosis from thrombophilia and hypofibrinolysis.

References

Balasa VV, et al.: Legg-Calve-Perthes disease and thrombophilia. J Bone Joint Surg Am 2004;86:264. [PMID: 15590848]

Glueck CJ, et al.: Role of thrombosis in osteonecrosis. Curr Hematol Rep 2003;2:417. [PMID: 12932315]

Herring JA, et al.: Legg-Calve-Perthes disease. Part II: Prospective multicenter study of the effect of treatment on outcome. J Bone Joint Surg Am 2004;86-A:2121. [PMID: 15466720]

Transient Synovitis of the Hip

ICD-9: 716.45

- ■ Essentials of Diagnosis
  - Benign; likely immune response to viral or bacterial infections a few days to 2 wk prior; usually unilateral
  - Two thirds of patients are boys aged 3–10 y
  - Increased synovial fluid in the joint produces pain; fluid is resorbed in 3–7 days
  - Physical exam shows hip in flexion, abduction, and external rotation (position of maximum capacity)
  - Ultrasound shows distended joint, >2 mm difference between joint space of involved hip versus opposite normal hip
  - WBC count and ESR are normal
  - Aspirate hip under fluoroscopy; will have high intra-articular pressure

- ■ Differential Diagnosis
  - Septic arthritis
  - Legg-Calvé-Perthes disease
  - Slipped capital femoral epiphysis
  - Juvenile rheumatoid arthritis
  - Acute rheumatic fever
  - Tuberculosis or tumor
  - Pain originating from spine (diskitis), knee (osteochondritis dissecans), tibia (toddler's fracture), or ankle

- ■ Treatment
  - Bed rest, NSAIDs; may use traction, with hip and knee partially flexed
  - Recurrence in up to 17% of patients; if symptoms recur, it is usually within 6 mo of the initial episode

- ■ Pearl

Key findings help differentiate this benign process from septic arthritis. The best predictors of septic arthritis are fever (oral >38.5°C), followed by elevated CRP, elevated ESR, refusal to bear weight, and an elevated WBC count.

References

Caird MS, et al.: Factors distinguishing septic arthritis from transient synovitis of the hip in children. A prospective study. J Bone Joint Surg Am 2006;88:1251. [PMID: 16757758]

Kocher MS, et al.: Differentiating between septic arthritis and transient synovitis of the hip in children: an evidence-based clinical prediction algorithm. J Bone Joint Surg Am 1999;81:1662. [PMID: 10608376]

Developmental Dysplasia of the Hip

ICD-9: 754.30 Unilateral; 754.31 Bilateral

- ■ Essentials of Diagnosis
  - The neonatal hip is relatively unstable, which may lead to subluxation or dislocation; lack of concentric positions for the acetabulum and femoral head may lead to dysplasia
  - Incidence is <1 per 1000 per year, less common in African American children and more common in some North American Indian tribes; increased risk in patients with family history, breech presentation, female gender, large fetal size, and first-born infants
  - Infant is asymptomatic
  - Physical exam shows positive Ortolani or Barlow test; in the Ortolani test, the hip is out and pops in with abduction and anterior force; the Barlow test is the opposite—the hip pops out with adduction and posterior force
  - Radiographs are not helpful in the newborn but become useful at 4–6 mo when the ossific nucleus of the femoral head appears; ultrasound may be useful but clinicians must be careful of false-negative results before 10 wk

- ■ Differential Diagnosis
  - Familial primary acetabular dysplasia

- ■ Treatment
  - Infants aged 0–6 mo: Pavlik harness may induce spontaneous reduction of the hip; a 1-mo trial is warranted
  - Infants 6–15 mo: perform gentle closed reduction under anesthesia followed by spica cast application
  - Children 15 mo to 2 y: open reduction of the hip is necessary, and femoral shortening may be required, followed by spica casting
  - Older children require significant surgical interventions to achieve and maintain a reduction of the hip; these vary from case to case

- ■ Pearl

Screening hip radiographs for patients with clubfoot are not warranted.

Reference

Weinstein SL, et al.: Developmental hip dysplasia and dislocation: Part I. Instr Course Lect 2004;53:523. [PMID: 15116641]

10

Rehabilitation

Joint Contractures

ICD-9: 718.4

- **Essentials of Diagnosis**
  - Contractures of joints usually occur following trauma, strokes, surgery, or as a progression of neurologic or arthritic disease
  - Contractures occur due to inactivity, uncontrolled spasticity, or iatrogenic immobilization
  - Lower extremity contractures compromise standing ability and may contribute to pressure sores on the heel
  - Hip and knee develop flexion contractures from sitting; elbow is prone to flexion contractures due to trauma
  - Joint contractures are examined by assessing both passive and active ranges of motion (ROMs) and comparing these to the normal ranges; in joint contractures, both passive and active ROMs are decreased

- **Differential Diagnosis**
  - Neurologic disease
  - Degenerative joint disease
  - Postsurgical arthrofibrosis
  - Post-traumatic injury
  - Postamputation
  - Adhesive capsulitis of the shoulder
  - Dislocation

- **Treatment**
  - Contractures can first be treated with physical therapy, bracing, or splinting; having a patient lie face down ("proning") will treat hip flexion contractures
  - Excessive muscle tone or spasticity must be treated aggressively to prevent contractures
  - Surgical releases are reserved for patients who have not responded to conservative management, for those with hygiene issues, and for instances in which surgery would improve patients' ability to ambulate, sit in a wheelchair, or to fit into shoes

- **Pearl**

Contractures are usually progressive and should be treated as soon as they are brought to clinical attention.

References

DeHaven KE, et al.: Arthrofibrosis of the knee following ligament surgery. Instr Course Lect 2003;52:369. [PMID: 12690864]

Issack PS, Egol KA: Posttraumatic contracture of the elbow: current management issues. Bull Hosp Jt Dis 2006;63:129. [PMID: 16878834]

Spasticity

ICD-9: 334.1 Hereditary spastic paraplegia; 342.1 Spastic hemiplegia; 344.0–344.9 Noncongenital or noninfantile; 781.0 Abnormal involuntary movements

- **Essentials of Diagnosis**
  - Condition in which specific muscles are continuously contracted; muscles show an excessive response to quick stretch
  - Continuous contraction can lead to stiffness of joints and shortening or contracture of muscles and may interfere with normal movement, gait, speech, and swallowing
  - Damage is normally localized to the spinal cord or brain, areas that control voluntary movements
  - Often associated with spinal cord injuries, multiple sclerosis, myelodysplasia, cerebral palsy, brain trauma and stroke, adrenoleukodystrophy, phenylketonuria, and amyotrophic lateral sclerosis
  - Generally, when all muscles in a segment of the body are spastic, the stronger muscles cause contractures
  - Symptoms include hypertonicity, clonus, hyperreflexia, muscle spasm, and fixed and stiff joints

- **Differential Diagnosis**
  - Positional contractures (hip and knee flexion, ankle equinus)
  - Peripheral neuropathies

- **Treatment**
  - Medical treatment is first line; medications include antispastic agents (ie, baclofen, tizanidine), antianxiety drugs, and benzodiazepines (ie, diazepam and clonazepam)
  - Physical therapy can be used to improve range of motion and help prevent shrinkage and shortening of muscles; there is minimal evidence for efficacy over the long term
  - Surgery may be indicated for tendon releases or lengthening
  - Osteotomy can be used to correct deformities

- **Pearl**

Botulinum toxin type A (BTX-A) as a therapeutic tool is being used; however, BTX-A to treat spasticity is off-label.

References

Criswell SR, et al.: The use of botulinum toxin therapy for lower-extremity spasticity in children with cerebral palsy. Neurosurg Focus 2006;21:e1. [PMID: 16918222]

Pin T, et al.: The effectiveness of passive stretching in children with cerebral palsy. Dev Med Child Neurol 2006;48:855. [PMID: 16978468]

Young RR: Treatment of spastic paresis. N Engl J Med 1989;320:1553. [PMID: 2725586]

Decubitus Ulcers (Pressure Sores)

ICD-9: 707.0

- ■ Essentials of Diagnosis
  - • Caused by a combination of poor nutrition, lack of sensation at pressure points, and decreased ability to move
  - • Result in lengthened hospital stay and cost, and delayed return to normal function
  - • Pressure causes anoxic injury from interference with blood supply
  - • A pressure sore can develop in 20 min in an insensate extremity that is not moved to relieve pressure (eg, comatose patient on a trauma board)
  - • Many different assessment tools are available for predicting pressure ulcers and for evaluating them; simple tests to determine nutrition are WBC count and serum albumin

- ■ Differential Diagnosis
  - • Surgical wound breakdown
  - • Cellulitis
  - • Abscess

- ■ Treatment
  - • Prevention is better than treatment
  - • Adequate nutrition is associated with healing of pressure sores; the prognostic inflammatory and nutritional index (PINI), which evaluates albumin, prealbumin, α_1-acid glycoprotein, and CRP level, is useful in predicting prognosis
  - • Many treatments are available for the local wound care of pressure ulcers
  - • Once skin breakdown has occurred, the wound-vac is quite useful, combined with debridement where necessary; surgical skin coverage by free or rotation flaps can be beneficial if the wound is clean and free of osteomyelitis

- ■ Pearl

Constant vigilance by all providers is necessary to prevent pressure sores.

References

Brand PW: Pressure sore—the problem. J Tissue Viability 2006;16:9. [PMID: 16505284]

Reynolds TM, et al.: Assessment of a prognostic biochemical indicator of nutrition and inflammation for identification of pressure ulcer risk. J Clin Pathol 2006;59:308. [PMID: 16752707]

Ankle-Foot Orthosis (AFO)

ICD-9: not applicable

■ Essential Features

- The AFO is one of the most widely used orthotics in orthopaedics
- Device is made of metal or polypropylene (most common), or a combination, and usually extends from the proximal tibia to just proximal to the metatarsal heads; it is usually open on the anterior aspect, and different models exist that can either allow dorsiflexion and plantar flexion motion at the ankle, or can totally eliminate ankle motion
- Dorsiflexion assist from springs can be included
- AFOs can be temporary and premade, or they can be custom fitted for each patient's needs
- AFOs may be prophylactic (to prevent injuries), homeostatic (to supplement function), or therapeutic (to treat problems)
- Thorough clinical exam of the lower extremity is needed to choose the best AFO for a patient

■ Essentials of Management

- Applications: foot drop, foot inversion, equinus from spasticity (ie, stroke, cerebral palsy), ankle arthrosis, ankle fractures, medial or lateral subtalar instability, ankle instability from weakness of the muscles (ie, polio, weakness or rupture of the tibialis anterior muscle weakness)
- AFOs can be used for patients with inadequate dorsiflexion, medial-lateral instability during stance (varus or valgus deformities of the subtalar joints), and inadequate tibial stability during stance, caused by weak plantar flexion

■ Pearl

The primary requirement is that the joint must be able to be passively positioned, as the orthotic cannot correct fixed deformities. Spring loading can be counterproductive in the spastic extremity.

Reference

Grissom SP, Blanton S: Treatment of upper motoneuron plantarflexion contractures by using and adjustable ankle-foot orthosis. Arch Phys Med Rehabil 2001;82:270. [PMID: 11239325]

Knee-Ankle-Foot Orthosis (KAFO)

ICD-9: not applicable

- ■ Essential Features
  - Indicated for patients with quadriceps weakness, hamstring tightness, or knee ligamentous instability, or for correction (with spring-loaded action) of flexion or extension contractures
  - Foot extension is used either for maintenance of orthosis position on the extremity or to correct concomitant foot-ankle pathology
  - It is more difficult to ambulate with a KAFO than with an ankle-foot orthosis (AFO)
  - Device can be fitted with a polycentric joint that can be adjusted, depending on the patient's clinical needs
  - Patients with intact proprioception may be able to walk with an unlocked polycentric joint KAFO

- ■ Differential Diagnosis

- ■ Essentials of Management
  - Hamstring spasticity is an indication for hamstring release or lengthening rather than a KAFO
  - Varus, valgus, anterior, or posterior knee instability: prescription can specify purpose of KAFO
  - Intact hip flexion function and proprioception, as is found in patients with polio and usually not in those with spinal cord injury, are necessary to utilize an unlocked knee mechanism
  - A hyperextension stop should be used in patients whose quadriceps function is stronger than their hamstring function, to prevent back knee (genu recurvatum)
  - Patients with a locked KAFO at the knee should be fitted with a drop-lock to permit passive knee flexion when sitting

- ■ Pearl

Due to their lighter weight and form-fitting shapes, polypropylene and carbon-fiber composite KAFOs are much more functional and, therefore, beneficial for patients with quadriceps weakness and knee instability than double-upright metal KAFOs.

Reference

Bakker JP, et al.: The effects of knee-ankle-foot orthoses in the treatment of Duchenne muscular dystrophy: review of the literature. Clin Rehab 2000;14:343. [PMID: 10945419]

Complete Spinal Cord Injury (SCI)

ICD-9: 806–806.39 SCI with vertebral injury;
952.0–952.9 SCI without vertebral injury

- ■ Essentials of Diagnosis
  - Characterized by a total absence of sensation and voluntary motor function caudal to the level of injury in the absence of spinal shock
  - Formal diagnosis is established after the period of spinal shock, which typically lasts 24 h
  - Patient has areflexia and a total absence of motor and sensory function below the injury level, and is often hyperreflexic after spinal shock
  - There should be no evidence of sacral sparing, and the bulbo-cavernosus reflex should be present
  - Root escape: when some root level function is regained at the level of injury; this should not be confused with the return of cord function (ie, a peripheral nerve [root] injury that has recovered)

- ■ Differential Diagnosis
  - Spinal shock
  - Anterior cord syndrome
  - Posterior cord syndrome

- ■ Treatment
  - Acute management: maintain systolic blood pressure >90 mm Hg; restrict fluids for 48 h; keep patient at 100% O_2 saturation; if injury is <8 h old, give methylprednisolone, 30 mg/kg over 15 min, then 5.4 mg/kg/h for 23 h
  - Prevent contractures by splinting immediately, especially elbow and wrist in the upper extremity
  - Aggressive pulmonary hygiene
  - Physical and occupational therapy
  - Psychological counseling

- ■ Pearl

Watch for autonomic dysreflexia especially in the patient with acute SCI.

Reference

Krassioukov AV, et al.: Autonomic dysreflexia in acute spinal cord injury: an under-recognized clinical entity. J Neurotrauma 2003;20:707. [PMID: 12965050]

Poliomyelitis

ICD-9: 045.9 Acute; 138 Late effects

- ■ Essentials of Diagnosis
  - • Viral disease that occurs secondary to infection with poliovirus, an enterovirus; since the advent of the Salk and Sabin vaccines, acute cases have become very rare in the US
  - • Virus affects anterior horn (motor) cells of the spinal cord, causing paralysis; variable numbers of motor cells survive, resulting in permanent paresis or paralysis
  - • Predominantly affects children; lack of muscle activity in the extremities results in reduced muscular loading and atrophy and failure of long bones to grow in length
  - • Problems include joint contractures and deformity secondary to unopposed muscular activity, scoliosis, and postpoliomyelitis syndrome—new neuromuscular symptoms that occur years (usually decades) after the acute disease has stabilized, producing symptoms of *new* weakness, muscular fatigability, general fatigue, and pain (cause is unclear but probably arises from aging [with motor neuron loss], overuse, and disuse)

- ■ Differential Diagnosis (For postpoliomyelitis syndrome)
  - • Muscular dystrophy
  - • Guillain-Barré syndrome
  - • Myopathy
  - • Amyotrophic lateral sclerosis

- ■ Treatment
  - • Initial phase treatment is supportive; aggressive physical therapy and orthotics during and subsequent to recovery phase are necessary to prevent joint contractures (eg, equinus, cavus foot, hip) and maintain residual muscle function
  - • Surgery may be necessary (ie, for tendon transfers in hand, joint contractures of hip or knee, or scoliosis correction)

- ■ Pearl

Prevention and treatment of postpoliomyelitis syndrome focuses on designing a lifestyle and exercise protocol that minimize disuse and overuse of muscle groups; this protocol will vary dependent on the residual function in each muscle group.

References

Klein MG, et al.: A comparison of the effects of exercise and lifestyle modification on the resolution of overuse symptoms of the shoulder in polio survivors: a preliminary study. Arch Phys Med Rehabil 2002;83:708. [PMID: 11884812]

Trojan DA, Cashman NR: Post-poliomyelitis syndrome. Muscle Nerve 2005;31:6. [PMID: 15599928]

Cerebral Palsy: Adult

ICD-9: 438

- ■ Essentials of Diagnosis
  - See Cerebral Palsy: Pediatric, for further details
  - Before the mid-20th century, few patients with cerebral palsy (CP) lived to adulthood; today, ~60–90% of children with CP do
  - 95% of children with diplegic CP and 75% with quadriplegic CP survive until 30 y of age
  - Adults with CP have many of the same health-care concerns that affect children with CP, as well as unique concerns of their own
  - Adults with CP have an increased incidence of cancer, stroke, ischemic heart disease, and breast cancer, which may reflect a lack of education or access to proper health care

- ■ Differential Diagnosis
  - Arthrogryposis
  - Familial spastic paraparesis
  - Static encephalopathy that occurs in adulthood (ischemic, infective, or traumatic brain injury)

- ■ Treatment
  - Physical or occupational therapy, or both, can often help improve quality of life, mobility, and overall independence for adults with CP
  - Use of proper orthotics and assistive devices can significantly improve quality of life
  - Medications such as oral baclofen and injected antispasmotics such as botulinum toxin can be beneficial
  - Surgery to release tendons (eg, adductor release), or lengthen tendons (eg, Achilles, hamstrings, iliopsoas, gastrocnemius) can improve function and hygiene
  - Patients with CP can develop scoliosis that may require surgery to prevent progression, improve ventilation, and improve hygiene

- ■ Pearl

In adult CP patients with impaired speech or mental retardation, every effort should be made to obtain a thorough history and exam. Family members and long-term care providers often can help clinicians understand the needs of such patients.

Reference

Zaffuto-Sforza CD: Aging with cerebral palsy. Phys Med Rehabil Clin N Am 2005;16:235. [PMID: 15561553]

Index